Intimacy: Living as a Woman After Cancer

Jacquelyn Elnor Johnson

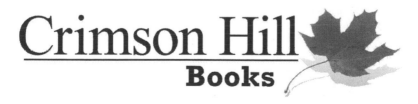

Crimson Hill Books

www.crimsonhillbooks.com

Copyright Jacquelyn Elnor Johnson, 1987, and Crimson Hill Products Inc., 2017

Canadian Cataloguing in Publication Data

Johnson, Jacquelyn Elnor

Intimacy: Living as a Woman After Cancer

ISBN 978-1-988650-33-3

1. Johnson, Jacquelyn Elnor. 2. Cancer-Patients. 3. Cancer-Psychological aspects.

I. Title

RC265.6.J64A35 1987 362.1'96994'00922

C87-094274-3

This book has been re-edited and added to by the author for this new 2017 edition.

This is a book about how real women cope – emotionally and spiritually as well as physically – with the challenges of living with cancer.

It is not intended to be used in place of professional advice, treatment, or therapy.

Cover and book design and formatting: Jesse Johnson

Cover Art: Sun Spiral by Galyna, via Stockfresh.com

CONTENTS

FOREWORD

If you live in Canada, the U.S., UK or elsewhere in the developed world, you have about one chance in two of being diagnosed with cancer in your life.

If you learn you have cancer, you have slightly better than the same odds of surviving for five years or more after diagnosis.

But what will the price and the quality of survival be?

Cancer threatens life, and it changes it. For those of us who live, our bodies and our relationships are forever altered.

Like other serious traumas, cancer attacks your sense of self, as adult, strong and competent. It weakens you and threatens your life and everything in it.

Cancer attacks women about as often as men, but the cancers women develop are more likely to affect the parts of our bodies that we believe define us as women or are directly linked to our sexuality. So, for women, more frequently than for men, cancer is a disease that threatens our lives and attacks our image of ourselves as people and as feminine, sexual people. These cancers, once considered to be a tragedy of advancing age, are striking younger and younger women. It's no longer unusual to find women as young as in their 20s and even in their teens with breast and gynaecologic cancers.

What happens after cancer? How do we cope with our losses? How do we rebuild our lives? And how do we, with our lovers and mates, tear down the walls cancer throws up around us and reaffirm our relationships?

How much truth is there to those horror stories of women deserted or rejected by lovers after cancer? These are just some of the questions I had as I started to create my own survival. I asked these questions of women, their mates, family members, doctors, nurses, counsellors and caregivers. Their responses form the backbone as well as the heart and soul of this book.

After I had cancer, I felt lost and alone. I wanted a lover to hold and comfort me. I needed friends to listen to me and I needed other women who had gone through the cancer mill and survived to help me sort through my feelings of loss and despair.

I was single then. I lived alone, with no supportive lover. Some friends could listen, for a time. Most quickly wore down. In 1979 and the early 1980s, I could find no other young woman who'd had breast cancer. So, I looked for a self-help book, one that would tell me women's experiences of survival. I needed to hear, from them, that life's possibilities, including affection and love, hadn't been cancelled from my future, however long or short it might be.

How do you tell a new man, a potential lover, that you don't have a right breast, I wondered? And when do you tell him?

How do you tell a man who wants to marry you and envisions the children you will have together that you have had a hysterectomy and have also lost part of your vagina?

How do you talk about how afraid of recurrence you are and how each clinic check-up is an agony of anxiety to a good and loving husband who, you fear, is being alienated by the topic of your health?

How can you face a scarred body in the mirror every morning after a shower, and still start your days feeling beautiful, confident, healthy and vitally alive?

There was no book to tell me how other women face these problems. So, I began to write the book I needed to read, beginning my research in 1980 and writing this book in 1985-1986. It was published in 1987, becoming a bestseller in Canada and going into two reprints.

Then the small publisher who produced it went out of business, and this book went out of print. For some years, friends and family have urged me to revive it and update it and now, 30 years after it was first published, I have.

Why now? It is because, re-reading this book just recently, the first time I have looked at it again for many years, it struck me that relatively little has changed in the cancer survival universe. The chemo drugs used, the surgery methods, the radiation techniques – all are very little changed, though we do use these in somewhat different ways. Our caregivers know more about cancers than they did; yet there is still no proven cause; no known cure.

The struggles of survivors, the feelings, the emotions, the pain – these are no different in 2017 than they were in 1987, or in any previous decade.

Today, we do know about the strength of the human spirit and how we react in times of trouble – what psychologists call "trauma." Much of this research has come about in response to the suffering of soldiers captured and imprisoned; not by studying people living with cancer.

The '90s also gave us a new name for people in and after trauma who are not doing well – they are suffering PTSD, Post Traumatic Stress Disorder.

In that decade and since, psychologists have also studied how people cope with trauma – that is, how they survive despite PTSD. Or cancer. Or any other life-disrupting event.

Though I wrote this book before these relatively recent breakthroughs in our understanding, in hindsight it is clear that women who had cancer and talked to me were living what experts would later confirm. They were, to put it into the psychologists' parlance, growing in resilience.

They were coping, in other words. They were inventing their own survival, day by day and moment by moment.

They were living with, and beyond, cancer.

This book was written and more recently re-edited by a woman who had cancer, primarily for women with cancer but also for the people who love them and care for them, from a practical and optimistic-realist perspective.

I write with the realization that individual women's needs are very different. There is no 'right' way to survive cancer. There are no correct answers to life's big questions; only starting points from which to form ways of living that can work for you.

I also realize that mates may be male or female. If you are a lesbian or transgender woman you may need to translate some of what follows to suit your life. While writing, I also kept in mind that some women live full lives without a mate, by choice.

There is no such thing as a typical woman with cancer. The problems of one may not affect another. We all deal with the threat of an early death, with changes to our bodies, with possible disability. But the problems of a rural woman who is 76 with lung cancer and is a widow are very different from those encountered by an urban student of 24 who faces having a colostomy or a mother of three who is 40 and has throat cancer.

There is no cure, yet, for cancer, nor for the havoc it causes. But there are strategies in coping that work for the women you will meet in this book. All of these women are real people, although most names and all actual identities are disguised because I asked women what name they would like to be known as in this book. Some chose their actual names; others prefer anonymity.

My aim here is to examine the problems women with cancer share from many viewpoints. In this way, this book is like a self-help group with occasional guest speakers from among the ranks of caregivers. We go around the room, with each woman offering her experiences, her perceptions, her insights on the questions having cancer has raised in her life.

Here are the stories of women who have survived cancer and who have reaffirmed themselves as complete women who work, who love, who live.

Here are the hurdles they faced, the love they lost and the love they've gained, both for themselves and for the people with whom they share their lives.

You and I are the still the same people we were

before cancer, but we have come through a passage, the door has closed behind us, and there is no way back to our former, pre-cancer selves. Cancer changes every aspect of life profoundly. As a result, we see our lives and ourselves differently. The people around us respond to us in different ways; sometimes in anger and confusion, at other times in compassion, and occasionally in an indifference it is difficult for us to fathom.

For women who are married or in a committed relationship, the quality of that relationship, the texture of its strengths and weaknesses are much the same, although cancer tends to strain already troubled marriages, sometimes to the breaking point. I have found that strong relationships (including marriages) become stronger and troubled relationships break down, following cancer.

The image of a woman with cancer reflects only the smallest minority. She is thought to be weak, elderly, alone and dying. But in this study, I did not find one woman whose life could so simply be summarized.

Possibly because of this image of a woman with cancer, many women are closet survivors who hide their pain, struggle, and eventual triumph like a dark secret. And, although each said she could not have survived without the love and support of at least one other person, each woman's survival is a story of grace under pressure ultimately achieved because of her own strength, faith and hope.

This book is not a basic information book on cancer treatment. It is not a workbook for solving relationship or any other problems. It does not offer answers because cancer, like a love relationship, is not a riddle to be solved.

This is a book about survival, about options and about what women's lives can be, after cancer.

Despite advances in surgery, chemotherapy, radiation treatment and the development of immunotherapies, in 2017 as in the last century, there is no proven cause for cancer and no proven cure. All the cancer statistics can really tell us is that cancer is widespread and it is affecting more of us, earlier in our adult lives.

All of us live, in some way, with cancer. No family is immune. How women live and cope and heal is the subject of this book. Ultimately, it is a book about being alive.

- Jacquelyn Elnor Johnson, Greenwich, NS, November 2017

INTIMACY

ONE

Why Me?

On one of the last hot days of summer, I set out to change my life.

"What will you do, way out there . . .?" my mother asked as I wedged more stuff into my car. "What if this isn't what you want?"

"I suppose then I'll try something else," I replied. Then I squeezed myself into the tiny space left behind the wheel and joined the trucks rolling west.

I felt great. Behind me were my surprised and doubtful family in the Pennsylvania city that had been our home for six years. During those

15

years, I'd earned my Bachelor's Degree while working as a waitress, a hotel clerk, a bookkeeper. Following graduation, I joined an advertising agency as a junior copywriter. But now, at age 28, I felt job-locked and bored. I wanted to do something new, in a new place, with new people.

All through that Labor Day weekend, I drove. There was plenty of time to contemplate the future. My new job would be teaching basic photography in the Journalism Department at South Dakota State University.

For three days teaching per week, I would earn a modest salary and full tuition for my own studies. In a year, I would have earned a Masters Degree in Journalism. In my fantasies, that degree, and my slim but growing portfolio of published writing and photographs, would pave the way to a staff position on a city newspaper. While earning my ticket, I would teach and learn and write in a small college town on the rim of the prairie. Ahead lay a whole new landscape to photograph, new friends, new challenges, new possibilities, fresh air, and maybe, with luck, a new love.

Three months later, early December. My prairie home is as picturesque as I had imagined, with tree-lined streets leading to the campus. Beyond town, the prairie ripples away to the west.

My colleagues are friendly. Most welcoming among them is the professor I work most directly with. Woody loves junk food, puns, the Mills Brothers, noisy musical clocks (there are 13 in his living room alone) and he is a great talker. The university is an agricultural college, I learn, with such exotica as the graduate program added relatively recently.

Graduate students are a rare breed here. We come from all over and we bond quickly.

The apartment I had rented sight unseen is large and sunny and, better still, my rent is now a third of what my old fourth-floor-walk-up was back East. The landlady, widow of a revered department head, enjoys hearing campus news and gossip and I enjoy the baked goodies she often leaves on my doorstep.

My students are more inspired by photography that I have any right to expect. My own studies are challenging. I miss my family and old friends, but I've made new friends and love what I'm doing. And I like this new, adventurous woman I have become.

While all the elements for happiness aren't yet in place, I can believe that they will be. The good things; the career, the right man, the baby I long to have will come. I must only be patient. For now, I'm optimistic, happy, moving ahead with my life.

And that slight tiredness, that strange weighty feeling? I hardly notice it. Natural enough, with so many adjustments to make, such a major life transition, I tell myself. Even though things are going well, so many changes so fast are bound to be stressful. My days are full. I feel as healthy as I ever have in my life. I'm fine.

What I did not know, did not even suspect, was that I had cancer.

One December morning I was showering and thinking in a hazy, early morning way about the day ahead.

Then my fingers stumbled over something hard. The day before there had been nothing there but the smooth underside of my breast. But that morning, there was something there, as large and hard as a peach pit.

I must be wrong, I thought. I'll forget about it, until tomorrow.

And if it was still there? Then, I decided, I'd go

to the university health clinic. I silenced the alarm bells going off in my head.

I put it out of my mind.

The next six mornings, the lump was still there. Hard. Unchanged.

Thursday, December 21. At the health clinic, I went through the routine. Signing in.

"And what is your problem today?" the intake clerk asked.

"Personal" I said. A knowing smile crept across her face. Among any student population, "personal" health problems are usually either venereal disease or pregnancy.

I was shown to the examination room and handed the usual skimpy gown. I waited. Eventually (in the time it took me to mark three of my students' final exams) a tall, very thin middle-aged doctor and a very young and shy nurse entered.

I said, "There's a lump. In my breast."

"Hmm," the doctor said. He picked up my chart, reading. Then he felt the lump.

"Perhaps we should have someone else take a look." He wrote out his referral to "a good man" at the clinic in town who, I would later learn, was also the area's only surgeon.

As I dressed, the intake clerk called the surgeon's office and made an appointment for the following day.

"Lots of women have lumps," the doctor said in parting. "Nothing to worry about. And Merry Christmas!"

I worried. It was a lump. I'd never had a lump in my breast before. It could mean . . . something awful.

I drove home.

I showered.

I dressed to go out.

Friends arrived and we went to the only fancy restaurant in town, to celebrate the end of the semester and a birthday.

My birthday, that day. My 29th.

As new friends offered a toast, I tried not to think about the appointment the next day.

"Try to be calm," the surgeon commanded. "We're almost done, now. Take deep, long breaths. Relax. Breathe slowly. Deep breaths."

I was near panic as I lay on the metal table, under hot fluorescents, all but my chest draped in green cloths. There was only a local anaesthetic, so I could feel the pressure of the surgeon's touch as he worked.

I tried to think about tropical beaches and the Christmas gifts I had chosen for family and friends, fighting the urge to leap up and run from the operating room, past the jungle of machinery, down the green halls, out into the winter sun.

"Okay," the surgeon said just when I thought I couldn't stand it any more. "We're though."

I sank back, consciously releasing clenched muscles in my neck and shoulders.

"How are you now?" he asked, taping a white dressing over the wound.

"Piece of cake," I said, attempting a smile.

"So, don't get this wet. No showers for a while. And don't worry. Probably nothing more than a lump. That's what 80 per cent of these lumps are. Nothing at all. Especially at your age!"

The lump was gone from my breast. I was sore, but all the worry and anguish were over now, I told myself.

The lab would test that small part of me and find absolutely nothing at all. Just another harmless lump.

Soon, classes would resume. The normal cycle of my days would begin again with the new year. I'd be back to my familiar self, back to work. The lump and the worry would fade along with the bruises on my breast.

I was so convinced I was just fine that I did not tell my family about the biopsy during our Christmas phone call.

On Boxing Day, I packed my loosest shirts and sweaters and joined friends for a week of cross-country skiing.

Only one person noticed that I seemed to be favoring my right side, that I seemed to lack energy. When she mentioned it, I said I'd had a biopsy, but it was nothing, really.

I remember how crisp the snow was; how clear and bright the stars were in a black satin sky. I remember how good the brandy tasted when we gathered around the fire after an afternoon outdoors. I remember dozing off during the ride home, feeling happy and relaxed and totally satisfied with this new life.

The phone was ringing as I unlocked my door.

It was the surgeon's receptionist. "Come in," she said. "Now!"

"But it's almost 4:00!" I said. "Aren't you about to close?"

But she'd already hung up.

It must be just to check the stitches, I thought. While applying lipstick and brushing my hair, I caught my mirrored reflection and the sombre expression held there.

For a moment, it seemed that I was looking at a young woman I had just recently met, someone I did not know.

"You have cancer," a voice whispered to the woman in the mirror.

Foolish thought. I recalled the surgeon saying: "For women under age 35, less than one per cent of breast lumps we take a look at turn out to be malignant."

One percent! Which left 99 percent odds that I was as well as I felt. So how could there be anything wrong?

This time, I was shown to an examination room immediately.

I took off my sweater and blouse automatically

and put on the green paper gown. The surgeon entered with a nurse. I searched his face to read an expression, but could not. His eyes were flat.

"It's cancer," he said. "You'll have to have a mastectomy. The sooner the better. I think it should be in the next few days. I'm sorry," and he turned and left the room.

I tried to speak, but there was no sound. I couldn't remember what I was supposed to do next. I couldn't seem to get the paper gown off.

The nurse found my blouse and helped me into it. I noticed she was crying, and idly, I wondered why. I felt vague, detached, airy.

My eyes didn't seem to be working and I fished in my purse for my sunglasses.

Then, somehow, I was in my car, stopping at a red light but I could barely make it out.

Another time lapse, and I was parked. On campus.

Not at the journalism building, in my coveted staff parking spot, but in front of the modern main building of classrooms and offices. It came to me that I was there because I wanted to see Nancy. Feeling stiff and very weak, I eased myself out of the car and went to find her.

24

Nancy Helgerson worked then as a state home economist, which meant that she advised consumers on everything from how to choose roofing to how to buy and use the best, most efficient microwave oven. In those days before the Internet, extension home economists served as consumer educators. Often, like Nancy, they also taught architecture and interior design students.

I hoped she would be at her desk, not in class. She was. So was her officemate.

I heard myself making small talk with Nancy and with the woman who shared her office, but it was another woman's voice, like a radio announcer in the background.

In my mind, I could hear: "I'm going to die. I could be dying, even now." That soundtrack repeated while somewhere, far away, women's voices chattered on about a ski trip.

Nancy suggested coffee, tactfully excluding her office mate and led the way to a conference room.

"There's something wrong, isn't there?" she asked as she closed the door behind us.

I told her. She started to cry. She came over to my chair and put her arm around me. I sobbed.

"You've got your car?" she asked eventually.

Did I? I tried to remember. "Yes . . ."

She bundled me into her car and back to her apartment.

She made dinner.

Later, we curled up with wine and giggled through an old Laurel and Hardy movie.

She made popcorn. We talked about clothes, men, great old movies, make-up, her brothers, my sisters.

Not once did we mention cancer. It was like being 16 again, sleeping over at my best friend's house. I wrapped the afghan Nancy's grandmother had made around me. She uncorked another bottle of Chablis. We toasted each other, friends, women in general. Later, I was able to sleep for a few hours.

The next day, I called my family.

My mother flew out. We met with the surgeon.

Mastectomy, he said, and then a year of chemotherapy. He also recommended that I have my ovaries removed. That would mean I would never be able to have a child and it would also mean sudden menopause, but it might contribute to my survival.

We could seek a second opinion, he said, but it should be done quickly. I didn't have medical insurance; didn't know who else to consult or where, or how.

My mind was clogged with fears; fear of dying, fear of living. But there was no time, the surgeon said. We must make decisions, now, choosing treatment that might save my life.

"What do you think we should do?" my mother asked the surgeon.

"Go home and pack your toothbrush," he said. "I can schedule you in for tomorrow morning at 8:00." I agreed to mastectomy and chemotherapy, but rejected the removal of my healthy ovaries and the hysterectomy.

Later that day. My mother had gone back to my apartment, alone. I waited for the sleeping pill to take effect, but it only seemed to make me more edgy. I paced the halls. My thoughts were vivid.

I'm going to die.

Even if I do live, what will there be to live for?

My body will be mutilated, deformed, ugly.

I may not be able to work.

I'll be half a woman.

What man will ever want to hold me, to make love to me, to take the chance on becoming involved with me?

How will my body nurture a child, if I can even conceive after chemotherapy?

"Are you scared?" the night nurse asked.

"Very scared," I said.

In the dim light of the hospital hallway, while other patients slept, she held me. She rocked me like a child. She was younger than me, but still she comforted me. I went back to my bed, but could not sleep.

I lay there, waiting for dawn. The longest night of my life.

Friday, January 5. I lay on a gurney. My hair was held in a paper cap; white surgical knee socks were on my legs. My period had started in the night, but I could not have a tampon, not in surgery. Instead, I wore a bulky and uncomfortable maternity pad.

I waited for the tranquilliser to calm me. "My hand is over my breast," I thought, watching the injection for IV. "It's safe."

With deft movements, a pretty nurse in surgical greens taped the needle in place and hung the bag. She worked quickly, not looking at me, not saying anything. I was just the object on the table, not a human being, not a woman, not someone who was terrified.

Then she left me, parked in the hall outside the operating room.

My hand is on my breast. They can't take it. They can't get to it. It will be okay...

There was pain. When I awoke fully, my mother was there, in my hospital room, and so were my father and youngest sister. It hurt to breathe. My right arm and hand seemed to be paralysed. I am right-handed. No one told me to expect this.

There would be more bad news, more jolting discoveries. The surgery was just the beginning.

As I recovered, I began to read everything I could find about cancer. I learned about suspicious symptoms, suspected causes and possible cures. I read of cell biology, and of what happens when a cell turns wild.

I researched alternative treatments, hospice care, reconstruction. I learned how to buy a prosthesis, ways to relax, how to make chemotherapy more bearable, who was doing what research and where.

Rather naively, I believed that to face a problem and then overcome it you must start with research to understand it. This is true. What I didn't know was that what I needed to know wouldn't be revealed in any book then available.

Then, as now, there was no shortage of books about cancer causes, treatments and possible cures. It's hard today to look at any media – newspapers, online, television news – and not find another post or story or feature about cancer in almost every edition.

This was also true back in 1979.

It was not until I got beyond the fear and beyond the biology and chemistry and started asked the more intimate and personal questions, such as "How will this change my life? How is one to live, as a cancer survivor? Where are the role models?" that I began to put my experience of cancer and treatment into perspective.

Over the next several months and then years, I came to see that cancer's most profound and far-reaching effects are not physical. Rather, they're emotional, relational and spiritual.

Cancer makes vast changes in how we view ourselves and in how we relate to those around us.

When my body was altered by cancer, the way I perceived my body, as comfortable, attractive, sexually desirable, changed. The way I saw myself, as young, strong, healthy, in control of my life, also changed. And so, the way I related to the people in my life and the way they related to me changed.

Possibly because these changes are so personal, often so painful and so hard to place next to any barometer, these are the topics that remain mostly overlooked in the cancer research literature and in the training cancer care providers (particularly surgeons) receive. Then, as now, empathy (except for cancer care nurses) is in short supply.

Cancer builds walls between people. Cancer is isolating, and the isolation can hurt far more than the treatment. Suddenly, you, the person with cancer, find yourself on one side of the wall, the sick side. Everyone else in your world is on the other side of that wall, the normal side.

Also on your side are other people, some of them terribly ill looking, others who appear normal, but they all sit with you in the waiting room, and all of you are aware that you are there for the same reason.

You can pretend you are in that waiting room, reading six-year-old copies of Oprah's magazine or *Reader's Digest* while a family member or friend is the one here to be examined. But this form of denial breaks down when a stern voice calls your name, usually mispronouncing it. Heads turn.

You gather yourself and dutifully follow, to another dingy cold room, another paper gown, another wait for another test, more probing, more uncertainty.

It can take a long time to get used to the routine and its discomforts. To connect that ugly word, "cancer," with your own name, to say even to yourself, "I have cancer" and "I belong here, with these other people who have cancer."

A few of my friends could talk about cancer. Most would not. As one said: "It's been three months now. Isn't it time you stopped dwelling on this?" Another thought I was being "morbid."

I persisted. I needed to talk. I needed insights.

Two male friends were marvellous ears-and-shoulders for me, yet for all their sympathy and compassion, they couldn't really understand why the loss of a breast meant so much to me.

They could grasp what it might be like to lose all sense of themselves as virile, desirable, masculine people after having cancer of the prostate or penis.

They could imagine the emotional pain of a colostomy or speculate about the adjustments required.

But, even though men do get breast cancer, my male friends could not really understand what the loss of my breast meant to me, as a woman and as a person.

Oddly, it seemed to me, neither could women who had had cancer years earlier and gone on to weather and survive other challenges and losses understand.

As cancer veterans, for them it was, as one said, "all in the past."

They did not really recall the depth of grief or the difficulty of finding a path out of the cancer maze to a reconstructed sense of self.

Perhaps that is because time heals. We tend to forget the intensity of labour, but never the joy of greeting a newborn child.

Pauline is a mother and grandmother, a former teacher and a volunteer for a cancer support group. I met her one lunch hour at the coffee shop next to the women's wear store she and her husband own. She is an attractive woman who looks at least ten years younger than she must be, as mother of three adult children, grandmother of five and a thirty-year classroom veteran.

I told her about my concerns. That all my relationships had shifted.

My mother now treated me like an accident-prone adolescent who'd brought "all this trouble" to our family. My father seemed to think I'd reverted to being a fragile and careless two-year-old.

My sisters wanted assurances that I was okay – by phone.

My current boss empathised, because his wife had died of cancer a few years before, but would future bosses, once they knew my health history?

I wanted marriage, I told Pauline.

I wanted my own family.

A child. A healthy child.

I wanted to work. I wanted love, passion, success, normalcy, happily ever after.

Isn't this what most women want? Not unreasonable desires, surely?

As I spoke, Pauline's look of dismay deepened, her green eyes reflecting my own unhappiness.

"I truly don't know what to say," she said after I had poured out my uncertainty and pain. "You're so young. When I had my mastectomy I was older, in my 40s. I was married to Ike. You'll have to come back to the shop and meet him. It was, and still is, a very good marriage. I think we are tremendously lucky!"

I pumped her for specifics, wanting to hear that the mastectomy hadn't mattered to their degree of happiness with each other.

It hadn't, she told me. And what about sex, I asked. Pauline described what many women would later echo. They ignored the surgery site completely, and often also the remaining, healthy breast.

Instead, Pauline said, Ike now touched or kissed her in other places, such as the back of her neck, her sides, her shoulders.

The sexual part of their marriage had always been good, Pauline said. Now sex with one breast missing was different but, she thought, just as good, or perhaps better than it had been before her cancer.

I also asked about their fears and how they had gotten through the time of diagnosis and treatment.

"We talked about it," she said. "And we just got through it. I can only assure you, it will happen. You will find someone, like Ike, who won't care about one breast. He will care about you. And who would want to marry any other sort of man?"

I went back to their shop to meet Ike. He was balding and effervescent, one of those people who everyone likes. He obviously adores his wife. She was right; they are lucky. It buoyed my spirits to meet them.

Another person who helped was the therapist my surgeon recommended, Cathy. She urged me to be fitted for a diaphragm, even though I had no need for one. She was right; just contemplating needing a birth control device cheered me tremendously.

I used to take it out of my bedside drawer and look at it, and feel more like a woman who could make choices about her life, including sexual choices, and less like someone (a prisoner, someone in a care home) to whom sexual expression is usually denied.

Cathy and I talked about relationships; how they start, how they grow, why they sometimes end. She helped me regain an image of myself as a woman and person who deserves to be loved; a person still capable of giving and receiving love. But she could not help me with my fears of a vanished sexual desire (the result of the chemotherapy drugs, I would later discover) that I feared might never return.

She didn't know how safe it would be for me to eventually attempt a pregnancy. She had no insights about how to handle the frightening first time with a new lover. She'd never counselled a woman with cancer before, she said. She had no idea what problems the disease and treatment cause.

At that time, there was no book written for counsellors working with people who have cancer, she discovered. There was also nothing about how young adults survive cancer, or other life traumas.

Cathy couldn't answer most of my questions.

Neither could I.

So, I returned to the source, women who have had cancer, and began what would be the first interviews for this book.

Based on American Cancer Society statistics, I learned there should be about 16 women in our prairie town who had survived cancer. I found seven who agreed to talk to me.

Usually, I discovered, they agreed to see me because they, too, sought information and reassurance. They asked about alternative treatments, relaxation techniques and general coping skills as well as what one woman called "assertiveness in relationships."

They, too, had already combed the library and pressed doctors and surgeons for answers and found there was little or nothing to answer their questions or provide reassurance. It was as if these issues mattered so little that no one had ever bothered to consider them.

Or, as one doctor I talked to said: "Just feel lucky you're alive."

That's what I, and other survivors, were being told, by (as I would eventually realize) caregivers who also had no answers and were protecting themselves with denial.

My conversations with women who are survivors (often evolving into a series of conversations) always raised more questions than possible answers. We weren't supported in asking these questions.

In them, I heard echoes of my own anxieties, fears, concerns, hopes and dreams; but found I could draw no patterns and reach no conclusions about how we as women cope with cancer.

I broadened the net.

My questions, and those women asked me, became the basis for a questionnaire. In it, I asked the basics of age, occupation, marital status, cancer diagnosis and prognosis and then moved on to more involved personal questions about how they and the people in their lives reacted to their illness and treatment.

"Did you contact a helping group, and did they help?" I asked.

"If you have children, how did you explain your illness to them?

"Has the cancer affected your love relationships?

"Do you dream about cancer or death?

"What were the big hurdles for you in dealing with cancer, and how did you overcome them?

"Do you feel differently about yourself now that you've gone through this experience?

"Does your mate?

"How would you react if you found that your best woman friend has cancer?

"What would you tell a daughter about cancer?

"Is your life worse, better, or about the same now?

"What do you foresee for your future?"

Then I placed an ad in the classified section of a popular women's magazine. Some respondents dutifully worked through the questions; others ignored them to concentrate instead on their own.

Reading the responses, it seemed to me that the earlier interviews had been a prologue.

In them, I realised, the real issues had largely been side-stepped. Though at times during those early interviews the women cried, we had generally hidden our deepest emotions.

We hadn't really talked about the toughest parts. Ironically, one of the questionnaire questions was: "Do you feel there is societal pressure to react to a personal disaster like cancer in a certain way, as in to 'Be brave and don't talk about it' or to 'Snap out of feeling sorry for yourself' or "Do you feel you have to constantly prove your wellness to the world now?"

The consensus was "yes."

The answers that came back were insightful, honest, considered and often, voluminous.

Some wrote reams, answering the questions in detail, then writing a few weeks or months later to add to their answers.

They wrote of their own need to read the answers of other women who they will probably never meet: "Let's make it as easy as possible for each other... by discussing it openly. I'm glad you're doing this book," one woman wrote.

While they wanted to read of other women's

experience, many women found it hard to reveal their own.

"Writing about this is extremely difficult. So upsetting," Donna wrote two years after her diagnosis. "I have yet to find anyone I feel I can talk to about the problems I face because of cancer."

"This was so much more difficult than I had anticipated," Per said in her reply. "I kept starting and stopping."

Sherry admitted that, at just two months after her mastectomy, she was probably attempting to answer the questions "too soon," that is, before she had come out of her initial shock and confusion.

Her answer was a howl of pain which she apologised for with self-effacing humor: "I am a writer by force, a women's crisis counsellor by choice, a mother by luck and a temporary hysteric by circumstance. I am anxious to begin working through this, coming out of this fog," she wrote when she requested the questionnaire.

It took her several months, and several attempts, to complete it: "I'm having a hell of a time with these questions," she wrote. "I need some kind of deadline. Feel that each of these questions must be handled daily. I can't wait to have answered these awful questions! Christ! I can't continue with this stuff today. I feel like a robot with some essential gear missing. I just am beginning to realise how shocked I still am."

Several women mentioned using the questionnaire to help them work through what was happening in their lives and how they felt. "It helped me to remember and also have a record of my feelings and thoughts," wrote a woman who kept the original and sent me a copy. "Thank you for this opportunity to share," another wrote. "It has helped me also to think about the past months."

Two women said they had worked through the questions during the first sessions of cancer self-help groups for women each had started in her community.

Donna, separated and living in a northern British Columbia lumber town, said the questionnaire was her first link with another woman who had cancer: "It is so very difficult for me to put my feelings into words... there are no groups up here to help so I am now starting one. Most people would rather help me forget it and don't know what to say. They lend their support, their sympathy, their pity, but when you haven't been through it, it's hard to imagine the emotions involved. Having to face your questionnaire really made me confront my emotions head on.

"Some days (many days) I would even avoid the room I kept the questionnaire in because it was so painful to take it out and look at it and think about the things it asked about. Now, it's done and I'm anxious to get it to you (and out of my sight) so I can once again approach these questions at a leisurely pace .... It must stir up a tremendous number of feelings in you to deal with so many intense emotions from your contributors."

It did.

Donna had pointed out something I did not realise until I tried to read through the completed questionnaires and look for the threads of our common experience revealed there.

I would read a few, then find myself dazed and unable to continue. Often, I would cry, not knowing why.

That was, for me, the second year after my own

diagnosis and a very difficult year in my life. In that year, I had a second mastectomy, both breasts reconstructed and chemo ended.

The women were right. The questions were awful to contemplate. For me, as well as for many of them, it was simply too soon.

Several times I would take out the questionnaires and try to read them, and every time I would be drawn back into the pain.

It would be another three years before I had made sense of my own cancer experience and could approach the questionnaires with the necessary objectivity.

"I think of you working on this," Sherry wrote,

"and that gives me courage." She added, "Keep at it! I think it will be good for you..."

She was right, eventually. As I hope it is good for all of us to work through and understand what has happened and is happening, rather than retreat into denial.

Cancer has happened; it is a fact. There is no going back to your pre-cancer self and life, so the only choice is to move forward, to create your own survival. It doesn't 'get easier' or 'go away' with time, but it does become integrated into who you are: human adult, woman, cancer survivor and perhaps survivor of other life events and all the roles in your life: daughter, sister, friend, wage-earner, perhaps business-owner, parent, volunteer…

For a long time, I could not face this project without reliving my own anguish and the same scenes of pain, frustration and disappointment women wrote or spoke of. It seems strange now that, during my early readings of the answers I had asked for, I felt the pain but was unable to recognise the triumphs.

When I read Sherry's response, I re-lived my own confusion and despair and self-doubt.

But she also wrote "the questions are healing therapy for me... I have met some incredible women who have beaten cancer. Some I have known for years and it is only now that they tell me they have had it... I am coming toward the light!"

Other women, further down the path toward integrating survivor into who they are and growing in resilience and acceptance, could say that their lives were better now than before their cancer because of the lessons learned in coping.

Barbara: "I wouldn't recommend my kind of experience to anyone as a growth experience, but I really like myself so much better now! I'm a much more positive person, I feel extra strength because I not only survived, but did it with grace and flair! I foresee only good things for my life now, but with the knowledge that if they should go bad (and some things will) that I can handle any situation."

That is personal power!

This new strength, this refreshing new enthusiasm for life was not the experience of the fortunate few. Most women had come to a more positive image of themselves as survivors.

"I am strong now."

"I still have some bad days. I get angry. I cry. But generally, I am happier now."

"I am stronger. I value living each day," are some of their comments.

These women had come to this point after a period of anguish. I did find a few deniers, women who seemed stalled, as one said, in "just not thinking about it."

But most women who answered had thought

deeply about cancer and their reactions and the reactions of others to them.

Because they had, they feel they are more in touch with themselves, and therefore with other people. They are more human, more alive and often, more connected to other people than they were before diagnosis.

One woman wrote a manual now given to women being treated at the cancer centre where she had her surgeries.

Another changed careers and now works to help recovering alcoholics. Several found the strength, after cancer, to leave unhappy marriages, change careers, move across the country or abroad, or finally follow another dream they'd been putting off. They realized that life is short.

In finding themselves after cancer, they had also discovered inner sources of compassion which they used to help others coping with personal tragedy.

Who are these women who answered that first questionnaire and the ones that followed it in 1986 and in 2017?

Most are either Canadian or American. Half live in cities. The youngest was 15 when I met her; the eldest 73, with most in their 30s and 40s.

One quarter consider themselves to be primarily homemakers, the rest are students, artists, office workers, professionals and trades workers of various stripes.

One woman, a single mother, struggles to get by on Mother's Allowance while she is learning a new vocation.

Another is an internationally-acclaimed author. One has been a nun for over three decades.

Several have started and run successful businesses. There is a school principal, a musician, a cook, a sculptor. Four are retired.

Twenty are happily married.

Seven had divorced before discovering their cancers, and four left their marriage or long-term relationship after cancer.

Three out of five have children.

Half of the 50 women had breast cancer, the rest had gynaecologic cancers, Hodgkin's or cancers of the brain, heart, liver, lungs or bone.

Among the women I talked to or heard from, five had had recurrences.

Women most likely to agree to answer the questions were from two months to several years post diagnosis, with the average being 24 months.

I have concluded that before two months, the experience is too raw, too overwhelming to talk about, and beyond about three years most women no longer have such a strong need to talk about it. Even though survival is a process, not an event, few women were willing to talk about their survival beyond three years. It could be that for them, the problems and doubts were either largely resolved, or, less often, denial tactics were firmly in place.

Life had moved on.

Beyond three years, women do talk about cancer, but by then I found they had often shifted away from a personal perspective and into a helping mode. Women at that stage often wrote of (usually volunteer) counselling they now do for other women who had recently learned their own cancer diagnoses.

There were six women who had never married, and 15 either widowed or divorced. But, though they were unmarried, they were not alone.

All the women wrote or told of someone (surprisingly often, this someone was a young child, even when the woman has a loving and understanding mate) who had given them the love and emotional nurturing they needed, when they needed it most. These women stressed that they could not have survived without this support, leading me to conclude that it may not be possible to weather cancer, or any other life-changing crisis, without the loving concern of at least one other person.

The women who share their experiences here are by no means intended to represent a controlled research group.

That was not my intention. They are women who voluntarily answered the questions about their relationships and their own feelings.

Not all of them answered all questions and some answers were evasive, possibly showing that their beliefs continue to evolve. It is possible that women having the most difficulty in adjusting to their new reality as cancer survivors would avoid participating.

After reviewing my answers from the first advertisement in the woman's magazine, I needed to reach more women.

So, I advertised again for women willing to answer a new, longer questionnaire, in a woman's magazine, a magazine for gays and a Toronto newspaper. And I asked everyone I knew who they knew who might be interested in answering my questionnaire.

Completed questionnaires trickled in.

Younger women tended to view illness and loss in a relationship context as well as in a personal context, while women beyond age 50 were more likely to see their cancer as a very private problem.

While many women seemed to interpret "intimacy" as "sex" and "sex" as, exclusively, intercourse, my definition of intimacy is much broader. Intimacy is familiarity with others and with oneself – innermost thoughts, feelings and concerns. Intimacy is connection.

For most women, healthy sex is a part of intimacy. So are body image, self-image, self-esteem, communication, trust and love. We are intimate with ourselves and with those we love, care about and spend our lives with.

In this book, you will not see the word "patient" except in this sentence and when quoted directly. We are women who have or had cancer, not cancer patients or cancer cases.

We are survivors, not from some point in the future, but from the moment of diagnosis.

This book is a place where we as women who are survivors share feelings and reach out to console as well as support each other as we try to come to grips with the profound changes cancer brings to our lives.

We live in Boston and Vancouver, Moncton and California and Coventry and many points between. We may be isolated physically but we are certainly not alone, as the women in this book attest.

I came away from this project with a tremendous feeling of admiration for the women I met, either in person or through their words.

Many had great difficulties in addition to cancer.

Some did not have the money they needed for treatment, or they lost their jobs, or a mate deserted or had his or her own major crisis at the same time.

Sarah had just entered adolescence and wanted desperately, as all teenagers do, to be accepted and to be popular. She succeeded, despite the loss of her leg.

Margaret has campaigned vigorously for major concessions for disabled workers at the conservative multinational corporation she works for, and she has seen real progress made because of her efforts. But she remains in the cancer closet herself because she fears losing future promotions to the ranks of upper management if her own health history is revealed.

Vervia struggles to remain positive in the face of her sixth recurrence in twenty years. For her, survival means living with chronic cancer.

All have found ways to face facts and accept, ways to change what can be changed, ways to put new meaning into their lives, ways to persevere if not overcome, ways to defeat anger, pain and bitterness. Ways to keep living.

They are truly valiant women, and I feel enormously privileged to have met them and share their stories. Some are triumphant, other cope in ways less spectacular, but all have defined their survival as so much richer than society tends to expect of people who had cancer.

Many of the women who agreed to talk to me or answer my questionnaire had not torn down the wall between themselves and the rest of the so-called normal world, but neither were they backing away from the wall or accepting it as unscaleable. Each in her own way and at her own pace was chipping away at that wall, giving it windows, building in doors.

The wall is built of ignorance. Society cements some of these beliefs into place; that cancer is contagious, for example, or that cancer is incurable and almost always terminal. Other beliefs, such as the one laying blame for cancer upon sexual misconduct or unhealthy emotional states are merely the current reincarnation of ancient ideas about what causes illness. Some of the bricks of misbelief are added to the wall by women with cancer themselves, using the cancer as an excuse for not trying to cope with life's random blows.

Before we can come to an understanding of what happens to women's intimate relationships with themselves and with the people in their lives, we must first examine the myths and prejudices that form the blocks of this wall.

INTIMACY

TWO

Breaking Down the Myths

The belief that cancer renders people so unattractive that no one, not even their mates, could possibly continue to love and live with them is widespread. It's also false.

Many people, even sensible, kind people, hold this and other superstitions or biases about people who have or had cancer to be truth.

These beliefs aren't logical. They are emotional, based in a mixture of fear and ignorance. People who hold these cancer myths to be fact have allowed their fear of the disease (and of people who have it) to overwhelm their reason.

The fact is that relatively few committed

relationships end after one partner has cancer.

Among the women I questioned divorce followed cancer diagnosis for only eight per cent, a finding that is similar to that of other studies.

These newly single women said their relationships had been troubled before cancer was ever suspected.

All but one woman felt that their relationships ended because of these long-term problems, not cancer.

The one woman who blames her divorce directly on her cancer said, "he invited me out of the relationship." Initially, she felt deserted, but now, three years after her mastectomy, she has come to see that "Cancer did me a favour! I'm rid of a weak man I spent twelve years of my time and health supporting."

Of these separated and divorced women, half have now built more positive love relationships. Ten women found new lovers and mates after cancer.

Like the myths we regard as truths about childhood, sex, marriage and many other aspects of life, cancer misinformation can limit the choices and the lives of people with cancer and all of us who live with them, love them or work with them.

No doubt you've encountered some of these prejudices, expressed subtly or directly and felt their sting.

You may have found these disbeliefs among friends, family, caregivers or even within yourself. Why do intelligent people, otherwise sensitive and caring people, believe these limiting and often contradictory myths?

Myths serve to comfort us and to fill in the gaps in our knowledge when there are no ready answers. They also shield us from painful or unpleasant truths, offering the pleasant illusion that we are in total control of our destinies.

The tragedies that can befall us in live – and there are many in addition to cancer -- we keep at bay by enveloping them in a fog of myth. But when we are threatened by crisis or tragedy, the myths that once served as protection from pain can work to alienate us from real comfort.

Myths can cause us more intense emotional pain than the object of our fears, at a time when we are most vulnerable to rejection and most in need of affection and acceptance.

Myths can also become expectations that constrict

our lives.

Myth: Cancer is always fatal

Cancer can be fatal.

Truth: Much depends on how soon the cancer is discovered, the type of cancer, the treatment chosen and the recovery of your immune system. There are cancers that grow and spread very quickly. Other types of cancer grow so slowly that they may be present for at least five years and as much as 20 years before being detected.

While it is possible to predict how quickly your type of cancer can grow and spread, no one can predict with absolute certainty how successful treatment will be for you, how long remission, a respite from disease and symptoms will last for you, or whether you will survive mere months of for years beyond diagnosis, because not enough is known yet about what causes cancer and why some people recover from cancer.

Researchers now believe what we call cancer is a group of diseases, probably with different causes. While there are treatments that are effective in reducing or eliminating some cancers, sometimes, for some people, no one knows with certainty what and who these are. There is no one proven and permanent cure.

And yet there are billions of people, worldwide, who are cancer survivors.

There are many factors that raise you risk of getting cancer, but no one proven cause.

For example, it is known that smoking contributes to lung cancer and that the rise in lung cancer in women (the second most common type of cancer among American women in 2016) is directly related to the increase of smoking among women in the past two decades. Yet, according to the American Lung Association, in 2016 more than half the women diagnosed with lung cancer never smoked.

Myth: Cancer is a disease of old age

Truth: Cancer is a disease of every age.

Cancer is the number one killer of children age 3 to 14.[1]

Once, breast and gynaecologic cancers were almost exclusively found among women beyond menopause (or age 50), but today, breast cancer is the major killer

---

[1]*https://www.cancer.org/cancer/cancer-in-children/key-statistics.html*

of women age 40 to 45. It is no longer considered uncommon for a woman to acquire a gynaecologic cancer while she is in her 30s, or breast cancer in her 20s.

Cancer is still most prevalent among people over age 50, but it can attack any of us, at any age.

Myth: Cancer is contagious

Truth: Cancer is not contagious.

When we do not know the cause (or cure) for a disease, it's human nature to conclude that the disease is contagious. It follows that segregating people who have the disease will protect the rest of us from acquiring it.

Until antibiotics became available in 1946, people with tuberculosis were segregated in sanatoriums where their 'rest cure' did help some to return to health. The fear of TB, and of polio lives on in people who can remember when thousands became disabled or died of these diseases every year. That segregation made sense, as it turns out.

We now know that TB and polio, caused by a bacteria and a virus respectively, are contagious in their infectious stages.

Today, our fears about TB and polio have simply been transferred to the diseases we cannot yet cure, such as cancer and AIDS. AIDS is contagious, but travels only through the exchange of body fluids such as blood, semen or saliva, not through the air.

Cancer may be in some way communicable, but not in the ways that a cold, TB or AIDS may be. Certain viruses are carcinogenic, meaning agents causing cancer, such as HPV, human papillomavirus, which is sexually transmitted and causes cancers of the cervix, vulva, vagina, anus, mouth, or throat.

Family members living with and caring for a person with cancer do not catch it.

If you are undergoing chemotherapy or radiation, your family cannot become irradiated or 'poisoned' by your treatment. Kissing or intercourse does not expose your mate to either cancer or the agents of your treatment.

Myth: Cancer is shameful

Truth: There is no reason for shame or guilt, any more than you would feel either shame or guilt if you were a survivor of another life trauma, such as discovering you have diabetes, or your child has a disability, or your town is destroyed by a hurricane.

Cancer is merely an illness.

Myth: Sex (either too much or too little) caused the cancer.

Truth: For most types of cancer, there's no link between a person's sex life and the risk of cancer. Nor does having sex after cancer treatment increase the chances of cancer coming back or getting out of control. But viruses passed from one person to another through sexual contact have been linked to some cancers. One example is Epstein-Barr virus, the cause of mononucleosis, also seems to increase the risk of certain types of cancer.

Viruses don't directly cause cancers. Instead, they damage your body on the cellular level, weakening these cells and sometimes even altering your DNA.

A cancer cell from one person's body simply cannot take root and grow in someone else. Not only are all cells fragile, needing the proper environment to survive, but the partner's immune system would detect the cancer cell and destroy it.[2]

And what about having sex during or after cancer

––––––––––––––––––––

[2]*https://www.cancer.org/treatment/treatments-and-side-effects/physical-side-effects/fertility-and-sexual-side-effects/sexuality-for-women-with-cancer/faqs.html*

treatment? A few chemotherapy drugs can be present in small amounts in vaginal fluids. You may choose to use condoms while you are getting chemotherapy and for about 14 days afterward.

Some types of radiation treatment require special precautions for a certain amount of time, too. Nurses at your cancer care centre will be able to describe these, specific to your treatment.

Some cancer treatments may cause harm to the fetus if you are or get pregnant during treatment.[3]

Sexual feelings and the need for touch, closeness, sharing and affection don't stop when you have cancer, or are beyond a certain age, or are ill.

Several women reported they felt sexually numb for months following surgery, but added that their physical feelings of desire did gradually return to pre-cancer levels (or better) as much as a year after chemotherapy or radiation treatments ended.

Myth: Cancer is war

Truth: Cancer is just an illness.

---

[3]*https://www.cancer.org/treatment/treatments-and-side-effects/physical-side-effects/fertility-and-sexual-side-effects/sexuality-for-women-with-cancer/faqs.html*

Despite this, you'll see such words as "bastion" and "arsenal", "army of doctors" and radiation "bombing" in what the media still call "the war against cancer." In describing our efforts to "conquer" cancer, the military model may be apt, except that for many readers this is not some distant battleground we are discussing.

This is civil war.

Our own bodies are the unwilling scene of attack and counter-attack. Two of the three most commonly used cancer treatments --chemotherapy and radiation -- are actually weapons of warfare (radiation is a product of World War II and chemotherapy chemicals were originally developed by American researchers to defoliate Viet Nam).

The war room model tends to appeal to caregivers, particularly male doctors, who can then see themselves as crusaders against the sick-cell foreign invader.

The military analogy may also be a positive one for some people with cancer, giving them the illusion of actively repulsing their cancer by imagining themselves to be the troops in white, marching bravely forth to attack and annihilate the dark forces of cancer within.

But for others, to whom war is literally hell, this analogy is monstrously offensive and can be psychologically damaging.

It's not pleasant to be invaded, less so to know that the invasion was helped on by our own supposedly treasonous immune system that watched the invasion and did little, or nothing, in our defence.

This is untrue. We all have cancers, likely many of them, throughout our lives. These are dealt with by our bodies, almost always before they're big enough to be detected. Occasionally, for reasons still not understood, our bodies aren't able to get rid of cancerous cells naturally.

It is likely that at some future time we will have a much better understanding of cancer on the cellular level. We'll know what 'turns on' or 'turns off' cancerous cells. We will be able to both reverse, and prevent, cancers. And leave behind today's blunt instruments of surgery, chemotherapy and radiation forever.

Myth: We already have a cure for cancer; it's being tested now. It will be available soon.

Truth: Sadly, we don't.

In the 1930s, it was confidently predicted that we would have found the "magic bullet", a cancer cure, by the 1950s.

In 1979, when I learned I had cancer, it was widely believed that the cure would be a certainty before the turn of the century. Millions of volunteers were raising billions of dollars to find that cure.

In 2017, despite the huge resources that have been dedicated to cancer prevention, detection and cure, there is no one, proven cure. Instead, we have come to view cancer as a manageable disease, like heart disease or diabetes. No cure, but you can live with it and live well, sometimes for many decades beyond diagnosis.

Myth: If you have cancer, you can cure yourself

Truth: If you have cancer, there's a lot you can do to help yourself survive better, for longer.

There are survivors and experts who claim that a 'fighting attitude' is the primary, or the only, factor needed to survive.

They say that if you want badly enough to live, you can cure yourself of cancer. But I believe that's like saying if you want to badly enough, you can cure your ADHD or your arthritis or your broken leg.

Others say that remaining positive with a can-do attitude is important, but it is only one of many factors involved in survival.

They point out that cancer, like any other health problem, is a physical illness causing emotional challenges and requiring both physical and emotional healing. I think this is true.

Most survivors I have spoken to agree that you must be assertive in seeking the best care and in giving yourself every health-promoting advantage in achieving your survival. This includes:

- Owning your cancer, not denying it;

- Getting treatment from the most knowledgeable, experienced expert in your type of cancer, at a major cancer centre.

- Working with the experts you have chosen to bring about your survival;

- Not hesitating to get a second opinion; knowing all you can about your type and stage of cancer and your treatment options

- Getting help from a team of experts in addition to your oncologist; realizing that no one person can provide all the types of help you need.

Your care must be designed to suit you, just as your treatments are planned in the most effective combination known to combat your type and stage of cancer; and

- Resolving to do all you can to heal your body and your mind. This requires searching within yourself to discover unresolved hurts, perhaps as long ago as your childhood, examining these ancient wounds and allowing them to heal. You need to understand and to forgive, not to let 'them' off the hook for hurting you, but to release yourself from these old chains that are taking far too much of your energy to maintain.

You cannot possibly be positive today if you still suffer for your past.

Cancer, cancer treatments and the way people around us react to cancer all deplete us physically as well as emotionally. It is at this time, when we are most vulnerable and most likely to be depressed, that it is necessary to strengthen ourselves for survival.

I do not believe that you can "fight" cancer and cure yourself, nor do I believe that "fighting" heart disease or TB or the flu will cure those illnesses, either.

However, I am convinced that taking a positive, assertive stance in getting the best physical and emotional care available and taking an active role in receiving the greatest possible benefit from that care can give the best possible chance for survival. It can also enhance your survival.

Myth: Cancer--caught early enough--is curable

Truth: Cancer is survivable and is sometimes curable, for reasons we still don't understand.

This is another belief that is both true and false. It is true that cancers caught relatively early -- that is, before they have metastasised (spread to distant sites in your body) can be treated with a higher rate of success.

What is misleading is that different types of cancer grow and spread at different rates. Many types are not diagnosed early because there are no symptoms until late in their development.

Cancers that have already spread are more difficult to treat.

The earlier cancer is detected, the greater the chance there is to stop it, or at least slow its progress.

Myth: People with cancer must be brave

Truth: Why? Cancer isn't a test. There are no medals of honour, no citations, no small golden statuettes for your mantle. No making the Dean's List or any list.

So why do we feel we must perform? Why not rage at the gods of outrageous fortune and cruel fate?

Why not rant, throw things, cry hysterically, pound the walls if we must?

Why do we people with cancer have to be so nice to everyone?

Why must we tiptoe around our doctors? [The truth: we don't. People with cancer are notorious, among doctors, for being among the angriest and most demanding of their clients.]

Why do we, the ones who are ill, have to become the 'strong' ones, ministering to our families and friends who look to us for comforting and guidance? We are the ones in the hospital beds, the ones throwing up in the bathroom, the ones trying on wigs and crying, the ones endlessly waiting for doctors to arrive, for a bed to be ready, for the test results, for if the next treatment works...

A part of this need to be heroines is, I think, tied to the pressure to be normal, even super-normal. After a crisis, we try very hard to 'act normal,' a contradiction. It is a way of both coping with the crisis and denying the intensity of the shock waves breaking up the structured calm of our lives.

We want to believe that if we 'act normal' we will *be* normal. Instead of working that magic, this belief works to deny us our true feelings, at a time when we are also denied almost everything else because our lives have been commandeered by appointments with doctors, nurses and several types of therapists.

You check into hospital, and you lose your clothing along with your identity. You can no longer chose when you will eat or what you will eat. There is zero privacy. Anyone can wander into your room, at any time.

Strangers come to examine, prick and probe. Treatment -- at the convenience of others -- now dictates your schedule.

Once out of hospital, you are warned that you cannot ever go too far from your lifeline of doctors, hospitals, clinics, the pharmacist.

For a time, you may be away from work as well as from your family -- an exile from adult normalcy.

Unlike most other people who are ill and in the hospital, you do not know that there will be one operation, one convalescence.

Your surgery may be exploratory; you may awaken to learn that you did not have the surgery you expected because your cancer is too widespread. Or that your surgery was more extensive than you expected.

Consider: who ever gives up so much with barely a whimper of protest?

After I awoke from my mastectomy, I waited in hope and agony for the lab report that would tell if the cancer in my breast had spread to the lymph nodes under my arm (because, statistically, the more nodes involved, the lower the chance of survival). Finally, a few days after surgery, while my parents and youngest sister were with me, the surgeon came with his report.

"I'm afraid it is not as good as we had hoped," he said. "There was lymph node involvement."

He went on to explain that my chances of living another five years was perhaps one in three. Maybe a bit better.

He would recommend a year of chemotherapy. And hope.

He was sorry.

While the surgeon was in the room, I only nodded, numb.

As he left, a great piercing wail of despair welled up from deep in my body, filling the room with the sound of raw anguish.

I saw my father shout something to my mother, who rushed from the room. Moments later, while I sobbed in great racking gasps, my mother reappeared with a nurse.

The nurse held a needle.

"You need this," I think she said. "Let's see your arm!"

I pulled away.

My parents urged. My sister crouched, terrified, in the farthest corner of the room. I still refused.

The nurse left.

My sister fled.

My parents sat, silently. After a while, to my very great relief, they went away.

Looking back now, I can see that it must have been awful for them. It can't be easy to bear seeing your child being told she might not live. That even after losing her breast, cancer will probably end her life within a few years.

I can understand my parents asking for a tranquilliser to calm me, perhaps also to calm themselves, to insulate us all, however briefly, from the ghastly news, after days of doubt and worry.

But in asking for that tranquilliser, my parents were also telling me that it was not okay to grieve, even though I had just received the most terrible setback in my life. It seemed they were repeating the message I heard so often in childhood: "Calm down!"

That is, be reserved, because we are reserved people. I must always be very brave, be strong, and never "give in" to my emotions. It occurred to me later that it is very strange that the sort of behaviour said to cause cancer (emotional passivity, the 'cancer personality' theory so prevalent among caregivers from the 1930s until well into the 1990s) was exactly the behaviour expected and condoned after cancer was discovered.

The idea behind the so-called cancer personality is that only a certain type of weak person, someone who can't control their lives, 'gets' cancer because of suppressed (unhealthy) emotions.

In fact, there is no cancer personality. But, I strongly believe, there is a survivor personality – someone who faces her cancer, acknowledges her true feelings, makes the best possible decisions based upon all the information and resources available and knows that 'acting' is not the way forward.

"Did you feel pressure to be brave?" I asked women. Of the 30 who answered, 21 agreed that there is pressure to be a trooper, while nine women said no one had expected them to be a "strong soldier."

It is liberating to honestly confront the problems life presents, without having to conform to anyone else's expectations of how you should be coping with the trauma you find yourself and your world rocked by.

Myth: People with cancer must be 'normal' as soon as possible

Truth: This isn't possible. There isn't any normal in the eye of the storm.

Yet there is an intense pressure -- both internal and external -- to return as quickly as possible to our usual routines, to "put cancer out of your mind," as one person recommended to me.

The problem is that everyone around you may assume you are right back to normal (as if all you had suffered was a cold that knocked you out for a few days) long before you really feel ready to resume your usual activities and responsibilities.

Also, you may be told that grieving should take a set period (one expert recommends that three months is "the healthy limit." Or you may read in a magazine that acceptance of your loss takes six months.

Ridiculous! Grieving takes as long as it takes, can't be rushed and is a very personal, individual and intimate experience.

It is common for survivors to feel like stubbornly determined, active 'fighters' during their cancer treatment. Then, when that treatment ends and they enter the "now we wait and see" phase, they run into trouble. It could be weepiness and aimlessness, when you can't eat, can't concentrate, can't seem to do anything but sleep. These are all normal during grieving but are also signs of depression. If this is how you feel, you may wonder if you are mentally ill. There is also the added burden of not getting back to 'normal' as fast as you, or anyone around you, desires.

What we must question is who set these time limits on grieving? For it is the grieving process you are going through -- grief for the loss of a part of your body, for its function, for your sense of youth, for your sense of personal attractiveness, for your former life, possibly for a job you have had to leave, for the worry and emotional pain your illness is causing to your family and friends.

How can 'they,' or any other person dictate precisely how long it should take YOU to mourn your losses? Only you can know this, just as only you can do the work of mourning.

Grieving is a gradual process that can take months or years. It is a passage that seems, at times, to have no end. As it does not. It changes in time, becomes less painful, less raw, less gut-wrenching.

There are times when the pain is worse, times when it is almost bearable.

But there comes a day when you realise that you can manage, despite your loss. It no long dominates your thoughts or ambushes you when you least expect it or dictates your life choices. The jagged edges, that awful raw pain, are gone.

They are replaced by a slight, bittersweet ache that

you notice less and less often.

When I asked women about the grieving they had done, some believed that they could (or should) skip grieving, but later discovered they were wrong.

Some did not grieve until long after their treatments had ended.

Others found that when they discovered they had cancer, they began to grieve for an earlier crisis or tragedy in their lives that they had never dealt with.

This is the nature of trauma. There can be flashbacks, to earlier times of loss and pain in our lives, earlier losses.

Their pain for the earlier event had remained buried in their personalities. That earlier loss was an unexplored inner territory that had to be discovered before they could begin to cope with the crisis of cancer.

For the first year after my own diagnosis, I was terribly brave. I gave myself high marks for my wonderful display of bravery, and smiled demurely when this Oscar-worthy performance was complimented. In the second year after diagnosis, I sank into a pit of depression, long after I should have been 'over it' according to several friends (none of whom had ever faced cancer or any other major trauma).

The pit seemed to have no bottom. I felt incredibly fragile, as if my body were made of bone china. I thought if I exerted myself, even moved suddenly, I would shatter.

I missed classes and barely made it to those I had to teach. I felt tired all the time. I felt sad. I had no desire to do much of anything.

Once I realised I was in mourning for my body and my self, I began to inch my way out of the pit.

Myth: Cancer patients don't die. They simply fade away

Truth: Cancer weakens us so that we have little or no resistance to other illnesses that end our lives.

We don't, finally, die of cancer. It is pneumonia, usually, that is the killer for people weakened by cancer. Or a stroke or heart attack (both can also be caused by chemotherapy).

Cancer is not a romantic sort of death, not the stuff we want to see at the movies. So, movie characters dying of cancer look a tad pale.

Remember Ali McGraw in *Love Story*? She appeared

week and ill, but not very much like a woman dying of cancer. In *Evita!* Faye Dunaway portrayed a beautiful woman who only appeared to need a good rest.

In *Terms of Endearment*, Debra Winger came closer to an honest portrayal of a woman trying to bring her life full circle, but in the scene when she says good-bye to her children, telling them to be brave but not that she is dying, she still only looks as if she has the flu.

Death from cancer is not nearly so sweet or so picturesque as the Hollywood version. So why romanticise it into a white death, the heroine pale, but stoic? Giving death the soft touch makes it more palatable for the rest of us. After all, no one wants to go through this pain, even if it is just a story, unless we have to. What we try to avoid knowing is that, sooner or later, almost all of us will be forced to deal with cancer.

Just as, at some point in life, almost everyone must go through a period of trauma: finding a way to live despite a tsunami, a hurricane, a volcano erupting, a war, loss of a loved one, an illness.

This romanticising of the terminal stages of cancer

not only insulates us from a possible future loss, it also trivialises that loss for those who have endured or are now trying to endure it.

People who are dying need to bring their relationships to completion, and the people surrounding them need just as much to resolve any anger, guilt, or ill-will as well as express their love and whatever else they have shared while there is still time.

We need forgiveness, and love.

When a woman is dying, she needs to tell those she loves how important they are in her life; she needs to hear that they love her and will miss her. Everyone needs to say the things that so often remain unsaid.

"Maybe mother did like you better, but it doesn't matter any more." "I forgave you long ago."

"I understand now why you married him/divorced him/moved to the coast/left the church..."

Most of all, what needs to be said sincerely is,

"I wish I could tell you how important your love has been to me, how much I admire you and how very much I will always love you."

There are also the practical considerations, such as

writing a will; providing for the future of young children when there isn't a mate or another parent or parent-figure, giving prized possessions to loved ones. Not dying and leaving a mess behind.

Women who are dying need to die as they have lived, that is, as themselves, not as the fading heroine in someone else's melodrama.

Cancer is not a sentence, not a judgement, not a punishment.

It is not something you somehow brought upon yourself.

It is not a metaphor for evil or sexual transgression or anything else. Something caused your cancer, but whether it was a sexually-transmitted virus, pollution, poor personal habits, hereditary predisposition or a combination of these causes and some still undiscovered, it does not matter now how or why you got your cancer. It is merely a disease, an organic disease of the immune system.

A disease which we do not yet understand and may never completely understand, but that isn't what is most relevant to your life.

When a cure is found, these myths will fall away and be forgotten, just as the myths surrounding TB and

Polio have faded from memory for everyone under age 70.

Until the time that we can prove what does cause cancer, what can prevent it, even what can cure it, no one can point the finger of blame.

If you blame yourself for having cancer, forgive yourself. Strip away the mythology, and its power over you. See cancer for what it is -- just a disease in cells that don't reproduce properly. Just an illness, much like many other illnesses.

Nothing more.

Nothing less.

You have cancer. It has changed you. Is changing you – not because of the illness but because of everything you are doing to survive the illness.

There is no path back to your pre-cancer life. There is only whatever measure of fulfilment and love and joy you can put into this day, this moment.

You grieve.

You cope.

You live!

INTIMACY

THREE

A Changed Body

One morning in January, 27 young adults wait for class to start.

I arrive, write my name on the board, apologise for having missed the first two sessions of this new semester and offer no excuse.

It's only a week after surgery to remove my right breast and most of the lymph nodes under my right arm and just a couple of days after my first chemotherapy.

I talk.

They listen.

At one point, I lean against the lectern, feeling queasy, head throbbing.

INTIMACY

Is this lecture making any sense?

Why aren't they asking any questions?

Will this class ever end?

I glance at my watch and am dismayed to see that we're only 15 minutes into the hour.

I continue to talk. They grow restless.

Finally, exhausted, I dismiss my students, but only ten minutes before the end of the hour. No one stays to chat. By then, I'm draped over the lectern, head pounding, hands sweaty, feverish.

But, I tell myself, I'm there. That's all that matters. Back to work, back to school, back to normal. Or so I keep reminding myself.

The truth is I'm in a state of cancer shock, like a small boat on a dark and angry ocean, being thrown about in the eye of the storm.

I can't eat, can't sleep and can just barely do anything else. My chest aches where there was once a breast, but now there's the red slash of a new scar, drains and stitches recently removed. Both my vision and my thinking are blurry.

Yet I must deny it all. No one must know.

Which is, when rationally considered, ridiculous.

In my fog of shock, confusion and grief, secrecy feels like the safest defense. I couldn't bear to be viewed as and treated like walking cancer, rather than the in-control person and woman I am.

Sympathy is hard to take.

Pity is intolerable.

Those first weeks after my first mastectomy, I put an incredible amount of effort into this charade, trying to convince everyone that over the Christmas break I'd had just a brief encounter with a minor illness. Something like the flu. Thus, the gray face and feverish look.

But getting over it now. Soon be fine. No worries.

To those few who know what's really happened, I joke that the surgery was "just a minor repair." While I draw boundaries and throw up barriers to protect myself, I also believe I'm protecting everyone around me. It seems vitally important to do this.

It's an exhausting one-woman performance for the benefit of myself, my intimates – family, friends, colleagues, students – my world. Body cancer denial and mind cancer denial of the facts: I live with cancer. It has spread. My body has changed, is changing and more changes are yet to come. There will be a year of chemo and, probably, more surgery. It is more than I can process.

And this is the essence of what is so challenging in the first moments, days and weeks of survival: at the very time when you must think clearly, logically and in problem-solving mode, gathering information to make life-changing and life-saving decisions and the marshalling your strength to act on these decisions, everything that is happening combines to weaken you in body and in mind.

Maintaining my one-woman performance of 'life as normal' took all the strength I had. This was the strength that I needed to direct towards my healing plan, except I didn't have one. It should have seemed obvious that I needed a plan, but in my post-anesthesia, post-surgery, post-chemo traumatised state, it wasn't. No one mentioned having a sensible, logical, realistic and well-considered healing plan, why you need one or how to create it in partnership with your caregiving team.

I had a surgeon who said, "Do this. You could get another opinion, but it isn't going to be any different than what I'm telling you, and there isn't time."

All, it turns out, untrue.

I should have challenged this but, frightened and vulnerable, I didn't.

Like almost every other woman with cancer back in the '70s and '80s, I had no caregiver team, no cancer center offering state-of-the-art treatment, none of the support services you find offered to women in cancer centres in the developed nations today.

Here's what I did have: a surgeon, who I visited once every three weeks for chemo, and a regular doctor, a G.P., who refused to talk about anything even remotely related to cancer. And, briefly, a therapist who had no experience of working with someone living with cancer.

So, in my chemo-addled, very frightened, worried and sleep-deprived state, I was trying to figure it all out; stumbling towards survival by seeking out other women who'd traveled this twisting path before me.

After the last student shrugged into her coat on that January morning, gathering her books and going on her way, I struggled to erase the boards. It didn't occur to me to ask anyone else to do this bit of classroom tidy-up, even though my body ached and my right arm no longer worked (I'd switched to doing everything, including driving and clumsy writing, left-handed). After straining to clean the boards, I sagged into the nearest student desk, sweating and breathless. Shaky. Exhausted.

I shouldn't have been there, but I had to be. I had to prove that cancer wasn't winning. I was winning because I was at work, doing my job, in control, earning my keep. Like any other responsible adult.

Trauma, fear, pain, the after-effects of surgery anaesthetics, chemo, desperate worry and lack of sleep can each scramble your thinking. Collectively, they make it nearly impossible to think clearly. But I either didn't know this or didn't want to know it. I was out to prove that cancer wasn't going to change my life, not in the least, not for one more moment.

It had attacked me, but I was fighting and that meant I was winning. I was going to keep winning.

The truth: cancer isn't warfare and I hadn't won; wasn't winning and was no battlefield heroine. I was the walking wounded, caught up in the grip of trauma and exhausted by denial.

Here's how it could have been so much less painful that bleak winter day. I could have levelled with my students, asking them to bear with me. I could have taught while sitting down. I could have launched a class discussion, leaving me to enjoy the role of moderator. That would have made a better experience for all of us.

The material on the boards, if anything needed to be presented there, could have been delivered as handouts created by the department secretary, who'd generously offered to help.

And there is one other thing I could have done that

would have been even easier. I could simply have taken off some of the six layers of clothing I was wearing and hiding under that day.

Shielding the scar and temporary prosthesis made from a wodge of pantyhose (it was too soon to get a 'real' breast prosthesis fitted), I wore an uplift padded bra, camisole, blouse, sweater and vest, all toped by my wool suit jacket.

The bra caused discomfort, but no professional woman goes bra-less. This is an absolute rule. I had to wear it. Somehow, it never occurred to me to remove the wire that made it an uplift bra, the wire that was now up against a new scar.

It seems ludicrous now to think of working in an overheated classroom while swaddled in all that cotton and wool. But I did not shed even one layer until after I got to the semi-privacy of my office. When it was time to teach my next class, I put my vest and jacket back on.

Encased in so many layers and pounds of cloth, I thought I looked professional and, above all, normal. In truth, I must have looked like I was wearing my entire wardrobe, like poor Anne Frank, walking to her secret annex in Amsterdam.

It would be almost three years before I could look at my body without hurling harsh criticism at what I saw as a maimed and ugly reflection of myself.

To my mind, I had an illness, I had surgery to remove the diseased body part, it was gone and so was that illness, I was having chemo for extra insurance, end of story.

But I never, ever looked at that body in the mirror.

It seemed I had to learn the hard way how dangerous denial is if you want to create a good and long survival.

It wasn't that I was suffering the loss of a favourite part of me. My breast and its neighbour had always been too small, in my judgement, to match my adult woman's body. My breasts seemed too girlishly high for me to wear plunging necklines or body-hugging sweaters, or any clothing I would then have defined as sexy, without feeling like a nine-year-old parading about in her mother's finery.

It was that same chronic dissatisfaction that many of us hold for our breasts, or our hips, or bottoms, or legs.

We look in the mirror, and instead of seeing fairness reflected there, we find our bodies are not enough to please us.

Hips are not slim enough, breasts not full enough, hair not thick and lustrous enough, body not tall enough, teeth not white enough. Eyes are too small, cheeks too broad, feet too large, waist too thick, noses too big or too tiny. One eye or one breast doesn't exactly echo the other *but it never does*. (This is true of everyone: here's the proof. Take an image of any person, and split that image into halves, vertically so that you have the right side of their face and the left side. Do this again, so that you have two right sides and two left sides. Put the two right sides together to form one face. Do the same with the two left sides. The result will be two photos of two people with distinct differences – not two identical twins. You could do this as a scissors-and-paper exercise, but it is much easier to do on your laptop.)

It is a completely unrealistic expectation that we will have perfectly 'regular' bodies and faces – yet these are what we see (digitally-altered) all the time in the media. The impossible ideals we are told we must strive for – or fail in the attempt.

Body image is the name given the map of our bodies we carry in our heads. If this map pleases us, it can be a boost to self-confidence and esteem that enhances our lives.

More frequently, we distort these subjective maps, sometimes bending and stretching our own images into shapes as warped as our reflections in funhouse mirrors.

Women are much more critical of their bodies than men, much more apt to have unrealistic expectations of what we should look like.

Multiple studies have concluded that most women don't like their bodies before cancer, so it is understandable that we have problems accepting our altered bodies after cancer. This negative body image is internalised before we even start school. For women, we believe that regular 'perfect' features are rewarded by love, sex, success, financial comfort and happiness, or so the societal myth goes.

For men, it is believed that the keys to all the goodies life has to offer rely more on who a man *is*, not merely what he looks like: intelligence, energy and ambition. Looks may help men, but aren't considered all that important. Points in appearance can be earned, if you are male, by being reasonably fit and well-groomed.

Women are judged, and we judge ourselves, on a much tougher scale, one that decrees that fitness and careful grooming are merely the starting points; that, in addition, we must be beautiful, and beauty is defined as physical perfection.

That our expectations for our bodies so rarely match reality does not lessen its hold on us. Or our harsh – often cruel – criticism of our own bodies when they do not match these beauty perfection myths.

The media, particularly movies, television and advertising, never tire of repeating these sex-typed myths. Our own vanity helps perpetuate them.

In real life, unlike most media portrayals, the pain of losing a part of your body and its function is multidimensional, complex and subtly intertwined with past and present happiness and accomplishment, at work, at love and in self-knowledge and self-acceptance.

Many of the women I spoke with and who answered my questionnaires said they felt mutilated if the cancer and treatment had claimed or altered a part of their bodies (as it does for almost every type of cancer).

Two months after her mastectomy, Sherry voiced the feelings of a woman who sees herself in the role of victim, a stance most of us take at some low moments.

She was anxious, confused, in despair and focused these feelings on the body she once liked but now found intolerable: "This feeling of corrosion: rotting, dark, unhealthy cells covered by very brittle skin. I feel so dried out. I look in the mirror and cannot see old Ms. Peaches and Cream. I no longer see youth. I see a woman who is beginning to look remarkably like her mother, with sagging eye-lids, with oh-my-God over-25 skin and with a lumpy, scarred body.

"I had a short affair with some fancy ex-princesses' make-up, but I felt like I was covering up the cracks. Never was terribly vain but now I'm angry to be cheated of a gradual ageing. My prognosis is good. But I feel like I am dying from the inside out, and I feel self-destructive, which is really bothering me. I don't feel I can fool anyone now into believing I'm beautiful."

While women who lost a breast commonly said they feel "deformed" or "mutilated;" women who had lost their uterus or vagina said they now feel "hollow," as if the core of their identity as women and as people has been removed.

Those who lost a limb, and have had to adjust to lost mobility and to the impossibility of hiding that loss, seem to have less difficulty coping with their changed bodies than women with the 'hidden' loss of a uterus, vagina, ovaries or breast.

"How can I cuddle my son now, without a breast?" Sherry asked plaintively. "How can he lean on a body that is so changed?"

For Sherry, and for the many women who find that without stimulation to their breasts it is much more difficult to become aroused or reach orgasm, the loss of a breast is more than a threat to physical attractiveness.

It is a threat to pleasure and success in both mothering and loving.

"It is hard to think of oneself as a sex goddess with one badly deformed tit and one half tit with nipple missing," one woman wrote. "Also, the nerve endings are no longer there and no longer function in a way that is sexually arousing."

Said another: "It is not so easy and natural to get turned on without breasts."

For women with gynaecologic cancers, the most common surgery is hysterectomy (removal of the uterus, cervix and a part of the top of the vagina) meaning that if the woman is in her child-bearing years, she can no longer have babies.

Intercourse can become difficult and painful. Even for women who have lost their uterus but kept their ovaries and most of their vagina, orgasm will be a diminished experience because it is the congestion of the uterus, that heavy feeling caused by blood coming from other parts of the body to the uterus (a small amount is changed to the lubricating fluid in the vagina,) that creates much of the physical feeling of arousal. Contractions of the uterus are also a major part of the physical sensations of orgasm.

Until recently, it was routine for surgeons to remove the ovaries of women with breast cancer, in the belief that the hormones produced by the ovaries stimulate the growth of any undiscovered distant colonies, or metastases, of cancer cells.

Untold thousands of pre-menopausal women lost healthy ovaries, and there were still some surgeons who urge all women with breast cancer to sacrifice their ovaries, before it was discovered that many organs, including the brain, heart and possibly the lungs, also produce these hormones.

Sex hormones also regulate other physical and mental functions in addition to the reproductive cycle.

Women believed doctors who told them to have an Oophorectomy (removal of their ovaries), sacrificing healthy ovaries for what they were told would provide an increased chance to survive.

Doctors knew, statistically, that more women survive breast cancer if they are among those who have their ovaries removed in addition to mastectomy.

At their doctors' urging, few women refused to give up their ovaries, even after it was discovered that only one in three breast tumours are stimulated to even faster growth by estrogen, the hormone produced primarily by a woman's ovaries.

A third of breast tumours tested are indifferent to estrogen and other hormones, and a third are suppressed by these same hormones.

It is now possible to test tumours to discover which ones are affected by the body's own hormones.

This test, called a hormone preceptor or hormone assay, is one you must request at the time of your biopsy.

If your tumour is stimulated by estrogen, having your ovaries removed may contribute to your survival. If not, their removal will be a needless loss, bringing about early, sudden menopause.

Since the discovery that only one in three breast tumours are affected by estrogen, most surgeons have advised against prophylactic Oophorectomy (unless the hormone preceptor result is positive.)

Why were so many women persuaded to give up their ovaries?

Was this medical guesswork?

Perhaps partially, although most doctors were working with the knowledge they had at the time, concentrating on saving women's lives and relatively unconcerned or completely indifferent to maintaining the quality of those lives after cancer.

Regard for how people can live with the results of

medical treatment is a concept that has been slow to dawn upon the awareness of the medical establishment. In the 21st century you will still find doctors (especially surgeons) who have little or no empathy for the women they treat; no understanding of what it means to a woman to lose a breast or her uterus or ovaries or any other body part.

Until the 1990s, there were very few studies on the quality of life following life-changing illnesses and accidents in the medical literature. Medical science, and therefore many doctors, still tend to view the normal functioning of women's bodies as pathological, meaning naturally harbouring illness, because our healthy functioning differs from the functioning of male bodies, taken traditionally by the medical community as the model of human health.

Even in the 21st century, there are still many doctors who diagnose and treat women as 'smaller men,' for example, as a rule prescribing medications that have been tested only on men in two-thirds the amount that they would for a male with no attention given to how the meds they use interact with female hormones or the female body's metabolism.[4]

----

[4]*https://beta.theglobeandmail.com/life/health-and-fitness/health/the-case-for-women-specific-advice-on-staying-healthy-as-theyage/article36201303/?ref=http://www.theglobeandmail.com*

Men who complain to their doctors of pain or discomfort are far more likely to be taken seriously.

Women are far more likely to be told that physical pain or discomfort, particularly in our genitals, are merely "to be expected because you're a woman," and prescribed tranquillisers.

Men are more likely to have heart attacks, yet women are more likely to die of heart attacks because women's symptoms (more usually neck, back or abdomen pain than chest pain and often more subtle) are less likely to be taken seriously, until it's too late. Men experiencing the symptoms of heart attack receive far faster and more aggressive treatment in hospital.[5]

If women get the impression that the medical establishment is just less interested in giving us appropriate care, who can blame them?

Our cultural ambiguity about the sexual parts of our bodies, particularly of female bodies, also must be held accountable. Our breasts and reproductive-sexual organs are the parts of our bodies most likely to develop cancer.

These are also, as philosopher Susan Sontag explores in **Illness as Metaphor,** the "embarrassing parts" of

---

[5] *Ibid.*

our bodies. As children, we are taught, except in the most liberated and enlightened families, not to talk about and never to touch our breasts or "down there."

When something goes wrong with our breasts and genitals, we do not give them the same loving attention we would give an injured eye or hand. Genital care is apt to be quick and secretive.

This is no less true of male genitals, which must, if anything, live up to even more exacting performance standards while usually receiving even greater criticism and less encouragement from their owners.

Kathleen V. Cairns, Ph.D., consulting psychologist and professor at the University of Calgary in Alberta, has specialised in the sexual rehabilitation of people with cancer since 1982.[6]

She told me of her own and other studies concluding that women who have had gynaecologic cancer are significantly more depressed and have a worse body image than either women who have had breast cancer or women who had a biopsy of a breast lump and learned they did not have cancer.

Gynaecologic cancer, cancer care nurse June Scruton told me, brings about a very different reaction among

[6] *https://www.linkedin.com/in/kathy-cairns-7a7a7a89/*

women than breast and other cancers. "Women who have cancer of the cervix or ovaries have already had pain and fear before their cancer was diagnosed. But for women with breast cancer there usually is no pain before treatment.

"Also, unlike breast cancer, a woman with gynaecologic cancer usually feels invaded in her most inner, secret self, at the centre of her femininity. With gynaecologic cancer, you almost always lose your uterus and usually a part of your vagina also.

"A vagina is something you use, as the birth canal for your children but much more frequently for lovemaking with your partner.

"A breast may be included in lovemaking, or you may ignore it. It is not so central to sexuality as a vagina and cervix."

As I watched June examine and interview, I noticed that with each woman she was very gentle, unhurried, caring and calm. I also noticed the women. All were extremely soft-spoken, all willingly answered June's questions and mine. None refused to allow me to sit in on their examinations. Some even apologised for, as one said, "being such a bother."

There was Greta, thin except for the rounded belly that is a sign of ovarian cancer.

She told me that her husband has been confined to a

wheelchair for over 20 years, and that she has supported their family by working at the post office. In addition to being the family earner, she also does all the housework.

When I asked her how she felt, she said she felt pretty good, although she knew the lab results she awaited would show that her cancer was terminal. She told me that she had once thought she would go on forever; that her husband, the ill person in the family, would die first.

Now, she said he would be very angry at being forced to move to a nursing home after her death.

The day I chose to follow June on her rounds was an average day at the clinic, she told me. The women I met are typical of women with gynaecologic cancers. Women with breast cancer come for treatment on another day of the week, June said, and on that day the atmosphere in the clinic is completely changed.

Although some women with breast cancer are depressed, they are not as depressed for as long a time as women with gynaecologic cancer, which has led June to conclude that these two cancers are in fact very different diseases, with different causes, affecting women in very different ways in both body and mind.

I found that the other nurses and doctors and that

caregivers at other centres agree with this conclusion.

It could well be that depression, which is deeply suppressed anger, does contribute to developing some cancers including gynaecologic cancer and that emotional healing must happen before physical healing can take place.

June Scruton takes this theory a step further: "I think there is a very strong mind-body link. Illness hits our weakest body part. I believe there is just so much we do not yet understand about this!"

Our feelings of shame are magnified when cancer attacks the colon, bladder or rectum. Now, in addition to the threat to sexuality, there are the potentially embarrassing problems of controlling odour and possible leakage.

Added to this is the fear that the appearance of the stoma, the opening for the bowel or bladder created by surgery, will show through clothing or, undressed, repulse a lover. [Before leaving hospital after an ostomy, you are taught how to care for your stoma so that odour and leakage are avoided. The stoma and catch bags are not visible under clothing, and you can cover your stoma and take off the catch bags before lovemaking.]

Women who have lost a breast or uterus or the function of their colons have the option of covering or disguising the damage cancer treatment has done with clothing.

Those who had cancer of the face, head, neck or skin cannot hide the physical changes.

Plastic surgery can help minimise the damage done to their appearance, but the period of waiting for the plastic surgery, or, more frequently, surgeries, can shatter self-confidence. Depending on where you live and your health insurance, it may also be unavailable, beyond what you can pay for, or both.

And plastic surgery can't always repair or disguise the damage.

Reconstructed body parts are never as authentic in appearance or feeling or function as the originals. Still, the reconstruction can do a lot to help a woman toward emotional recovery.

When a woman has cancer of the blood or lymph system (leukaemia, Hodgkin's) there is usually no specific physical loss caused by the cancer.

However, there are very specific losses caused by chemotherapy or radiation. Almost everyone who undergoes chemotherapy suffers the most obvious one, thinning or loss of their hair.

"You really don't know how important hair is, how much it is a part of your personality, until you lose it," Marti wrote.

Cathy, who lost her breast in her early 30s, said that when she saw her hair falling out, she cried. Of everything that happened during her cancer experience, "that was the most traumatic point."

Terry Fox is the marathon runner who lost a leg to cancer and then ran half way across Canada to raise money for cancer research, stopping only because his cancer recurred.

During his heroic run, he told one Canadian Broadcasting Corporation interviewer that for him it took more courage to face chemotherapy than it did to run 26 miles (43 km) a day with one leg.

Chemotherapy and radiation are miserable. The only plus side is that no one suffers from all the possible side effects, and some people are spared most of them. Some can be eased by medication and by relaxation techniques.

Some of the side effects of chemotherapy and radiation treatment gradually fade or reverse after treatment ends. Others can be permanent.

Here are the most common ones:

- Nausea, vomiting
- Diarrhoea, constipation
- Headache, earache, body aches, cramps

- Brain fog, confusion
- Fatigue
- Bloating, weight gain
- Loss of appetite, weight loss
- Fever
- Dry mouth, loss of taste, change in taste and sense of smell
- Insomnia, night sweats, bed-wetting
- Reduced vaginal lubrication, decreased sexual desire
- Anxiety, depression
- Thinning or loss of hair, including public hair
- Jaundice
- High blood pressure
- Suppressed immunity, susceptibility to infection
- Acne, skin rashes, dry and itchy skin, skin sensitivity, especially to sun exposure

Marti, a single mother of two who was told she would not survive because there was a tumour growing in the memory area of her brain, did live, did retain her memory and has raised her children.

Despite her strength and courage, she described herself during cancer treatment as "a bald, young, sexually needy woman who looks like Frosty the Snowman" because of the steroid drugs that are part of her treatment.

Wrote Mary Ann, a successful sculptor: "Before the cancer, I liked my body. I felt sensual, young at 45 and looking forward to old age. I expected to live a long life. Now (at 46) I'm a one-breasted, bald, fat old woman."

More than any other change, loss of their hair leaves women feeling that they have lost their youth along with their looks.

Bald men can be considered attractive, healthy, virile. Not so for bald women.

Several women said that when they lost their hair, they felt they were losing their identities. Throughout human history, when the objective has been to humiliate people; as slaves, in prisons or concentration camps, or to strongly encourage them to conform as in the military, their hair is cut very short or it is shaved.

One solution to thinning hair or baldness is to wear a wig, but women say wigs are only a partial solution. Other women opt for a collection of head scarves and hats.

Marti is a woman who looks hard for her silver linings.

She wrote that wearing a wig allows her to "be a

blonde one day, a redhead the next" which she enjoys, but "to be able to reveal my baldness to other people, I mean other than my family, was and still is frightening to me.

"For instance, when I meet a new man, and think about being intimate with him and the possibility that he would see that I am bald. I had to face the fact that making love would be uncomfortable with my wig on. And it might fall off or be pulled off in the process!"

Marti resolved this awkward problem by telling her potential lovers more about herself and her needs long before the decisive moment, and learned that by explaining her needs an opportunity was created to ask about the man's needs or fears.

It helped, she said, in getting to know the man better and in feeling closer to him before they had sex.

"I want to feel comfortable and open enough to accept his requests. Perhaps he would ask me not to remove my wig during intimacy," she wrote. "My other choice is to wear a scarf, gypsy style, which looks great with hoop earrings and can be tied tightly enough to stay in place."

Some women, like Marti, had reached a point of being somewhat comfortable with clothing and prostheses to disguise the physical damage caused by cancer and treatment. It isn't ideal, but they can live with it, for now, during treatment.

Others still feel they are now inadequate as women, saying:

"I'm mutilated,"

"I'm fat because of the steroids I took,"

"I'm so ugly now"

"I hate having to hide!"

Sadly, their attempts to appear 'normal' make them feel dishonest.

"I'm a fraud," said one. "Everyone says I look fine, but underneath I look terrible"

Feeling that she now impersonates "a complete woman" eroded her self confidence and hindered expression of her sexuality.

Other women told of the difficulty of finding clothing that fits or did not reveal a scar or ostomy appliance.

Cheryl, who had always been athletic and enjoyed swimming, still did not own a bathing suit a year after her mastectomy.

"I just don't know where to get one," she said. They're widely available, at big-city department stores, specialty boutiques, by mail, online.

But Cheryl couldn't bring herself to go and pick out a new suit. So, she didn't swim any more. For a while, for that matter, neither did I.

One Saturday a few months after my mastectomy, I went swimming with a male friend. Because my suit had a padded bra, I wore the sponge prosthesis given to me by an American Cancer Society volunteer. It was tucked into the bra cup of the suit, but not, unfortunately, sewn in because I had only one.

I dove in, surfaced in the deliciously cool water, and then was horrified to see the prosthesis floating away. I lunged after it and went underwater to shove it back in place, desperately hoping that no one else had noticed.

When I looked around for my friend, I noticed with great relief that he had just gone off the high board. Other people (there were only six in the pool that day) seemed not to have noticed either.

Many months later, when I could recall this incident and find it (mildly) amusing, I asked my friend if he had seen my float-away breast. He had, and we could laugh about it, but that day at the pool he had kindly pretended not to notice.

It shouldn't have bothered me, but it did.

I didn't go swimming again until after my breast was reconstructed. Really, I should have, because swimming is the best gentle exercise there is for regaining strength in arms and chest muscles after a mastectomy. I was just too embarrassed to swim in public, even though I knew I should, and could. No one was staring at my chest; not one cared. But I did.

Several women unconsciously developed odd compensations for their missing body part to try to 'look right' to the world.

For a few days after my mastectomy, I tended to hold my numb and almost useless right arm tightly to my side, sheltering it and protecting it. I didn't notice how this upset my family until my mother commented.

"Stop that!" she said one day in irritation. "It makes you look like you're handicapped!"

Which, at that time, I was. I was also permanently changed, but the people around me could not bear to be reminded of this.

If I continued to protect that arm, to not exercise it and not try to make it useful, I wasn't going to get beyond being handicapped. And I wasn't going to let other people around me forget it.

"My husband tells me I have this bad habit," Cheryl said, "when I take my coat off, I kind of shrug and readjust my prosthesis. He says, 'You've got to watch that!' I'm getting it lined up. I don't even think about it! But it really bothers him!"

Also, after mastectomy it can be tricky to shave under your arm if the armpit is numb. Feeling usually returns although it can take as long as a few years to feel normal again.

[In the meantime, if you are more comfortable with your armpits clean-shaven, you should do it very carefully. It may be easier to use an electric shaver or a depilatory.]

After mastectomy, it also helps to be aware of your posture. There is a tendency to slouch, compensating for the lopsided feeling because, until you get a properly weighted prosthesis or have reconstruction, the weight of your missing breast is absent.

For a while, I found I had to make a conscious effort to sit up straight and push my shoulders back. But there was also a benefit to this enforced good posture. Walking tall eased the neck and shoulder ache then and after reconstruction. It also helped me feel more confident, more in-control. Eventually, better posture – standing tall and proud -- became a habit.

All of us go to remarkable lengths to protect other people and ourselves from our losses.

Many of us can't bring ourselves to state our needs, feeling we don't deserve satisfaction of these needs now; even such a seemingly simple desire -- actually, a right -- for privacy in a changing room.

Another woman still goes to the Y to work out and swim, but she changes in the toilet cubicle, rather than in the locker room, because she believes the sight of her stoma might frighten younger women or female children who happen to glimpse her nude.

We impose these restrictions upon ourselves.

Most of the comments on using clothing as camouflage, or on the difficulties of dressing, came from women who'd had a mastectomy. "If you dress right, no one really knows," Joan wrote. For her, "right" means, "never going bra-less and not wearing V-necks. I wear a lot of loose blouses now and I like blouses with two breast pockets to hide any difference."

Donna, 32 and separated from her husband, had two mastectomies. At the time she wrote, three years after her first mastectomy, she was looking for a new lover and a new job and still working to accept her changed body.

"At times, this seems challenging and exciting, but more often extremely depressing," she wrote.

The problem she kept returning to in her reply was her attempts to hide her body: "One thing I've noticed about most people who have just found out about my mastectomies is that they tend to stare at my chest. Those few people who can refrain from doing this spare me a lot of pain and embarrassment.

"There is no woman's clothing made for women without breasts. I cannot wear clothing with darts in the bodice. I cannot wear sleeveless clothing, because of the scar. All low-cut or plunging necklines are out. All bandeau tops, sundresses and bathing suits with built-in bras. All sexy lingerie. All out. All a thing of the past."

Probably Donna could wear those clothes evicted from her closet, or at least most of them and look great.

My point is that after cancer we tend to exaggerate and we also tend to misread other people. That exaggerated self-interest and loss of logic is a normal part of grieving. Gradually, along with acceptance, comes a sense of perspective.

Donna has progressed to seeing herself as a challenged, not victimised, woman: "I feel very mortal after having had cancer, but that has made me all the more keen to enjoy my life while I have it!"

She is one of the women who are aware that they use clothing to hide, and although it may anger her or cause remorse, Donna and thousands of other women continue to live with their disguises in place and continue to work, to love, to do all, or most of the things they have always done.

While talking to women and caregivers, I heard of women whose attempts to hide themselves and their pain are much more extreme and limiting. This is not grieving; it is emotional illness.

Several women and a few counsellors told of knowing women who never leave their homes.

In every story, the woman is young, rather shy, a wife and mother who worked in her home before her cancer and now refuses to leave home for any reason.

I was assigned to visit a woman like this (in my role as a Cansurmount counsellor) but after our initial contact, she refused to talk to me. I cannot say why such a woman would find life as a hermit in the midst of her family less painful than donning whatever disguise she needs to venture out in public.

Women who answered my questionnaires did tell of new inhibitions that limit their behaviour and reinforce feelings of guilt and shame, such as avoiding their reflections in mirrors, always undressing in the dark, never allowing children or mates to see them nude, showering in the dark and wearing a bra and prosthesis over a mastectomy scar or panties to cover a stoma to sleep in, under pajamas or a nightgown.

Many women told of still not looking at their surgery site, even when caring for their bodies, for months after surgery.

Cheryl would not let her five-year-old daughter see her undressed following her mastectomy, although before that they had often enjoyed baths together: "She knew I went to the hospital," Cheryl explained. "We told her that the doctor had to fix my breast. Tammie did see the scar once, when I had just come home. I had on something, a nightgown, and you could see right through. She came into our bedroom. You could see the stitches, you know, the railroad track. She thought that was neat, but that was all we said."

That the "fixed" breast had been removed was never discussed with the child. She was not included in her mother's grieving, or told that her mother was seriously ill.

Some women do allow their children to see them as they are after cancer, and every woman who had been open about the cancer and her changed body said she felt it helped her and her children cope.

They felt their willingness to talk about their feelings of sadness and loss, while also reassuring the child that she was loved and would always be loved and cared for, helped them and their children accept and adjust.

"Where is my breast now?" Cheryl asked as our interview ended. "I think about it. What did they do with my breast? Do you have any idea?" Several women asked this question.

A part of their body was gone. It had died, yet there was no memorial for it, no funeral. It was simply gone.

"Your breast went to a lab, for testing," I told Cheryl. I didn't add that only a small sample of the tumour is needed for the lab work; the rest of the tissue removed from your body goes to the hospital incinerator. At the time, it seemed to console her to know that her lost breast could help in research, possibly in some way leading to a cure. A lab technician herself, she needed to believe in the power of research.

"That makes me feel better, if it's going for science," she said softly. "I've got my eyes willed, you know. They can take whatever parts they want, but I hope no one wants an extra breast."

She laughed then, relieved. "Somewhere, my breast is doing some good!"

INTIMACY

FOUR

A Changed Self

Cancer is a death in the body. It is also a death of the spirit. A death of a part of yourself.

As with any death, there is the need to mourn. But we live in a cancer-denying and death-denying society, where there is generally little support given people who are bereaved and mourning their losses.

At such a time, the greatest comfort is a kindly ear and shoulder. A friend who will listen and console without judging; someone who can allow you to grieve, at your own pace, someone who knows you, knows you need to mourn, and knows that eventually, your sorrow will mellow to acceptance.

It can be difficult to find such a kind and empathic

listener, when everyone is urging you to "just hurry up and get better."

"Be glad you're alive!" the people in your life are thinking, and some of them are also saying this. Yes, you are alive. But your breast is gone. Or you have lost the ability to speak or the ability to control your bladder or you can no longer walk.

"So, stop dwelling on it!" they may say. "Isn't it about time you got over it?"

There is no 'getting over' cancer or any major life trauma. It isn't a scratch that heals quickly, leaving no trace. You may very much want to get on with your life, may have been putting a tremendous effort into acting like you are getting along but you aren't, and you can't.

What you can do is move through your cancer experience and, eventually, beyond it. It isn't ever easy. It isn't as fast as you or anyone would want it to be.

Just after diagnosis, during treatment, just after treatment ends…these are still likely to be times when getting beyond cancer seems impossible. Not when it still takes every ounce of energy and all the will power you can muster just to get out of bed and get dressed each morning.

"Cheer up!" your well-meaning (but tactless) friends

and family may say. "You've got to fight this thing!" But why do you have to fight illness? Wouldn't it be more productive to join forces with wellness?

"You're going to be just fine!" they say. They can't know this. No one can. No one, including the doctor who 'gives' you X months to live, can know this. YOU can't know how your cancer experience will play out, until it does.

But will you ever feel fine again? How can you, when feeling good was a part of your before-cancer self, someone you just vaguely remember having been?

And now your with-cancer self is never without pain, both the discomfort and pain in your body, and the anxiety and other emotional pain.

Fact: you are grieving, for many losses: of your sense of yourself, as a healthy, strong person; as an attractive person; as competent and in-control of her life, as still young and fully alive, as strong, as someone with opportunities and options.

Grieving is not a defined state. It has no set boundaries, no exact start or finish. Like other intense emotions, we do not all experience grief at the same predictable pace.

There are stages of grieving from the initial shock at diagnosis to denial, depression, anger, guilt, fears and feelings of helplessness and, for some, bargaining with God.

These stages in the grieving process are eventually resolved, but we do not march through them in lock-step order, neatly ticking off the anger box, for example, before moving on to guilt or bargaining. It simply doesn't work that way.

Grieving, whether it is for the loss of a part of our bodies and the function of that body part or following the death of a very much loved and missed person or due to any of the many other life traumas and losses there are, is a journey of risk and pain as well as self-discovery.

In this journey, the destination is known, but there is no map and no information on either the terrain ahead or the distance to be travelled.

At times, it may seem there is no compelling reason to even make the trip.

And, while caring friends and family may offer comforts along the way, ultimately there are no travelling companions. A bereaved person, grieving a death in herself or the death of a loved one, must travel this road alone.

You may think you are the only woman who has ever come this way, ever penetrated this thorny wilderness. It can seem that no one has ever endured these hardships and uncertainties before.

The loneliness, that sense of being cut off from the rest of the world, can be very painful.

You may even think you are lost, that you are out of control, that you are driven by emotions so powerful that you must be losing your mind.

That you'll never stop crying.

Meeting other women who have had cancer, particularly women who have had the same type of cancer and similar treatment and are close to you in age and lifestyle can help you see that your mourning behaviour is not so bizarre and certainly not insane.

Knowing that they, too, felt such anguish, such intense rage, such seemingly bottomless sorrow and hearing that, with time, they came to the end of their journey of mourning can help you realize that the time will come when you, too, can feel good again, about yourself and about life.

That is not to say that grieving eventually just evaporates. There is no time when we can say, "It is over. Job done," because it never is absolutely, completely over. There will always be the physical changes in your body. Always the memories of your before-cancer body and your before-cancer life.

And possibly also regrets about what you did, or did not do, in the past – to live a healthier life, make better choices, be kinder to yourself, see 'the signs' of illness sooner…as women, there is no end to what we can blame ourselves for.

The missing part and its missing function, the scars, the lingering echoes of treatment and side effects will always be there to remind you of your loss. And within, you will always carry the essence of having grieved and healed.

Your loss, your recovery and the coping skills you learn along this cancer survival journey are part of the new woman you are becoming.

This renewed sense of self, as woman, as survivor and even as heroine, evolves as you are grieving.

But let us go back to the beginning.

First, there is the physical grieving.

Your body mourns.

It may be difficult to eat, because you feel as if you are being strangled, and food tastes oddly metallic or like mushy cardboard (a common side-effect of chemo and some other cancer drugs).

It may seem that you can't quite catch your breath.

Tears come easily and often, sometimes seemingly for no reason.

You feel terribly weak, as if you have a bad cold or

the flu.

There is a feeling of vagueness, of being unfocussed, of just wandering around, wondering what to do next, and why (a side-effect of chemo, radiation and a symptom of grieving).

You may feel like a robot, continuing to go through the motions of your days, serving customers or clients, supervising staff, preparing meals, caring for children, doing all those tasks that keep life going (like cooking and housekeeping) while all the time feeling like an empty shell that has been set in motion.

All these feelings are usual for people who are in shock. Learning you have cancer, even if you suspected the diagnosis, is very much like being hit by a truck.

If you had been in an accident, you would be kept quiet and warm. The ambulance would come. Attendants would care for you and reassure you while you were being rushed to hospital. There, other people would take over, marshalling all the wonders of medical technology to do whatever it takes to save your life.

A woman who has just learned she has cancer needs the same total attention and care, because she is in the same state of shock.

She, too, needs to be consoled, told that help is on the way, that she will be cared for.

She, too, needs immediate care for shock. But no ambulance rushes to the scene of diagnosis.

Sherry and her husband were already grieving the death of his father when they learned that she had breast cancer. It was during the funeral that Sherry slipped away to a pay phone to hear her biopsy results.

During the sermon, she whispered the news to her husband.

After the funeral, while Sherry and Bobby struggled to hold themselves together until they could be alone, Sherry's mother-in-law announced to everyone who had gathered at her home after the funeral that Sherry had cancer.

She remembers running from the house, running crazily down the street in a strange city, running and crying.

"Midway through my run I realized that I was not Ali McGraw [in the movie *Love Story*], that I had cancer, that I had to go back and face that roomful of strangers, that I had to face my husband, that I was in big, serious trouble."

She found her way back and she went to bed until

the next evening when it was time to leave for the airport and her own home.

Sometimes, her husband laid next to her, warming her and consoling her in his embrace.

At other times, she huddled there alone, knowing he was nearby. And sometimes, she held and consoled him. But they did not talk about it; not then, and not on the flight home.

"When I was sure it was cancer, I just wanted to leave my body," Sherry wrote. "I just floated away. It was very hard to come back."

As the numb confusion of the first hours after hearing a cancer diagnosis begins to subside, there come the doubts about the diagnosis.

Couldn't the lab have mixed the slides?

Couldn't there have been a mistake?

It's true that mistakes in diagnosis and lab report mix-ups do happen, but this is rare. It is much more common for women to believe such a mistake has been made. "I can't possibly have cancer," we all think. "Not me!" This belief, which may be held only in passing or which some people continue to hold for years, is called denial.

June Scruton, R.N. is a nurse-clinician [now retired] at the Gynaecologic Cancer Clinic, Henderson

General Hospital in Hamilton, Ontario. I asked her how many women with cancer want to believe that the lab has somehow made a mistake in their diagnosis.

"Most," she said. "It's a very common belief. They aren't blaming us, or the lab technicians. They are saying 'Oh, I'm hoping it isn't me. It can't be me!'

"Just recently, we did have one woman who wanted to see her pathology [lab work] for herself. She needed to be sure.

"I took her down to the lab, and the pathologist showed her the slides.

"He said he was only doing it because this woman is also a nurse, but I would have fought for any woman who wants to see; who had to be sure.

"I can understand that. I'd feel the same way, if it was me!"

Once that nurse saw her slides and saw that they matched her lab report, she could stop denying her diagnosis and begin making the necessary decisions about her treatment.

But very few women are lucky enough to have an understanding advocate like June Scruton.

Very few have the opportunity to see the evidence of cancer for themselves.

For a time, denial, psychological anaesthesia, may be a positive response to temporarily postpone the pain, until a woman is ready to face it. But denial that goes on for too long is avoidance, and ultimately it is destructive.

"You see constructive denial in a woman with cancer who's given a grim prognosis but chooses instead to focus on the grain of hope, saying 'If only one out of one hundred people lives, I'm going to be the survivor,' " Jay Lefer, Ph.D., a New York psychoanalyst, said.

"This belief may in fact help her to survive. A destructive example of denial would be the person who refuses treatment because she won't believe she has cancer. It's terrific to hope even if there isn't a lot of reason to, but it's terrible to deny that you're sick at all."

Why terrible? Wouldn't it be much less painful to ignore it all?

I talked about this with the close friend of a woman who has had cancer of the liver for several years and, to the amazement of her doctors, has survived.

Her family claim she has never suspected the truth about her illness. She was told she was in hospital "for observation" and later told her radiation treatments were for a relatively minor digestive ailment. Friends were warned not to reveal the truth. The family could manoeuvre this illusion partly because the woman's daughter is a nurse, and her treatments took place at the hospital where the daughter works.

Why have this woman's family and friends gone to such extremes to hide the truth, I asked?

"Because," the friend said, "We all knew Mabel is a worrier. She always has been. Even hearing the word cancer would kill her!"

And doesn't Mabel know that radiation is used to treat cancer, I asked the friend? Doesn't she suspect the true diagnosis?

"Oh no. She isn't one to read much, or even watch the news. She has never suspected anything at all. She's really much happier this way!" the friend said. "If she knew, she'd be dead by now."

The family and friends of this woman truly believe that their lies have saved her life. Perhaps they have.

There are some people who send unmistakable signals to caregivers and family that they do not want to know their true diagnosis or prognosis, or that they do know but cannot bear to talk about it.

That is their right.

In her classic book **On Death and Dying**, Elisabeth

Kubler-Ross, M.D. told of a woman who had read everything in the hospital library about cancer. This woman probably realized her cancer was advanced because of what she had learned about it in her reading, but she never talked about it, never asked any questions.

One day, she asked her doctor if she had cancer, but before the doctor could answer, she immediately interrupted with a story about her grandson. The message, clearly, was "I know as much as I can handle. Don't tell me what I cannot bear to hear!"

It may be that Mabel is like the woman Dr. Kubler-Ross treated, needing to deny her cancer or at least not talk about it.

But it could also be true that Mabel knows very well that she has cancer and wants to talk about it, but can't because everyone around her has thrown up a wall of silence. If that is so, she must be wondering what else they are lying about. And she must feel terribly alone.

One of the dangers of prolonged denial -- avoidance -- is being cut off from sources of consolation and comfort.

Another is that in denying pain, we may deny our other emotions; anger, joy, fear, love, desire, sadness as well as happiness.

Turning to stone is a defence that, for a few hours or a few days, can provide a mental breather. It can offer a time out, allowing a chance to get used to the awful truth and get ready to act.

Time to get another opinion, to look for alternative treatments or get to a cancer centre, to arrange for childcare if needed, to re-organize your schedule. It is also a defence we may return to many times for a brief respite when there is more bad news: when the cancer is more widespread than expected; the surgery was less successful than hoped for or the cancer has recurred.

Most of us are pushed out of the oasis of denial after only a day or two.

Doctors may stress the need to act quickly (seldom true. Most cancers are slow-growing).

Or they may say the opposite, giving a let's-just-wait-and-see message (standard for some types of cancer) that nurtures the seeds of fear, as Sherry's doctor did.

"He suggested I wait for a lull in my work schedule," she recalls. "I left his office knowing I must create a lull immediately!"

Sherry now believes her fast action (she got a second opinion) saved her life, but the loss of her breast sent her into a depression she wondered if she'd ever overcome.

"The trouble isn't that my breast is gone," she wrote two months after her mastectomy. "The trouble is under the skin. I feel unhinged inside. I feel raw and separated."

Annie, who was also 31 when she discovered she had breast cancer, wrote, "I felt set apart from everyone else. No one could really understand what I had gone through. And I felt old, because I had a disease one normally associates with old people. I know better now, of course, but at the time, who thinks rationally?"

None of us do.

Feeling ill, alone, and overwhelmed with the changes the diagnosis is bringing to our lives and the fears it is causing, we feel tired, depleted, empty. Desperate.

This feeling of terrible tiredness, this malaise, is a classic symptom of depression. It is also a known side effect of chemotherapy, radiation treatments or prescription painkillers.

With this powerful combination of physical and psychological triggers, it is understandable that women would describe many losses beyond the loss of a part of their bodies, among them loss of energy, ambition and sexual desire. (There is no more effective turn-off than pain, anxiety and stress).

It is also not surprising that during this period of

malaise, we can turn wistful eyes to our former, before-cancer selves.

We were happier then, we tell ourselves.

We were vital and fulfilled and useful and needed and kinder people.

We worry that the "younger" more carefree and happier woman we were is now lost forever. This belief can persist even after returning to all our normal activities and responsibilities.

Many women said it was not until their usual energy returned, which for them meant many months after radiation or chemotherapy treatment had ended and surgical wounds healed, that they were able to shake off their conviction that their lives were permanently diminished and that they may be dying.

A Harvard study published in the journal Nursing Research reached much the same conclusion.

The researchers discovered that depression among women with breast and gynaecologic cancers continued beyond the treatment period when there were lingering physical problems.

The intensity of a woman's depression after cancer treatment paralleled the number, and intensity, of her lingering disabilities.

They also found that women who had gynaecologic

cancer experienced more intense depression over a much longer time period than women who had breast cancer.

One explanation, according to the Harvard researchers, is that losing the ability to reproduce is a more profound loss than loss of a breast.

But they also suspect that the decline in hormone production following hysterectomy which brings on sudden, early menopause produces physical triggers for prolonged anguish and depression. [Depression is also common after natural menopause].

In other words, depression after menopause is not entirely emotional. It is triggered by the presence or lack of certain chemicals in the brain.

One of these chemicals, these researchers believe, is estrogen, the hormone produced primarily by a woman's ovaries.

A few women who had mastectomies mentioned the peculiar aching of the breast that is not longer there. This is phantom pain, common and frustratingly difficult to treat and to live with, after amputation.

Achiness around the healed wound may not be phantom pain but a permanent after-effect that is more noticeable when you are tired or before a thunderstorm.

It happens because scar tissue is less elastic than the tissue it is replacing and this sensitivity seems to be intensified when you are tired or during stormy weather.

If you have had a mastectomy, you may also notice that your scar site is achy around the time of your period each month.

Women also told of feeling terribly dependent, which they resent. It is as if they had been returned to babyhood, some said.

"Now, my family treat me like a child," Hannah told me. "I no longer work and they won't let me do anything at home. After dinner, I used to always do up my dishes. I like to do the dishes; have the kitchen looking nice. But now, my husband or my son say, 'You go on, sit down, rest.' I don't want to rest. I rest all day. That's all I ever do now."

She reached for a tissue and cried quietly. "I know it's terminal. But they thought I wouldn't live until February. Here it is July now. Sometimes, I think my family is just waiting for me to die."

In the depth of depression, many women think of death. Many plan for it. Some even wish for it as an end to their misery.

In her first letter, Sally, a nurse, described herself as "a woman who is coping with cancer." But her questionnaire answers showed a different woman, one who sees her cancer as only the most recent in a series of life disasters. Sally is pretending to cope, at a terrible psychic cost.

She is 49, a skilled operating room nurse, respected and liked by her co-workers. She is also the mother of two adult children, one a doctor and the other an architect.

On the surface, Sally is a survivor who has carried on with her life and who now counsels and inspires other women with cancer. But Sally also has been married, for 31 unhappy years, to an abusive husband.

She feels she cannot leave him: "I have no great desire for a long life. I look on my disease as an 'out.' It was only through a series of accidents that my family found out I was seeking medical advice. I flatly refused to have surgery, but pressure from the surgeon (calls to my home) and pressure from my children (instilling guilt) forced me to back down. I resent that they were able to manipulate me in this fashion.

"I live with my husband to enable me to save money to pay for my funeral. I have started giving my children anything of value I have, things I think might be meaningful to them.

"I have no goals, no priorities. I've tried to shut myself away from friends and family, and am succeeding quite well. I don't want them to get too dependent or concerned about me. I might let them down by dying. I guess now I'm not much of a woman or much of a person."

This is Sally's private face.

In public, which means with her children and at work, she puts on a happier mask.

"I maintain a positive attitude, certainly not the attitude I really have. That I keep to myself. My life is the same now, after cancer. But now, all I think about is death and planning towards that end. That's my future."

Only a few women would admit to considering suicide as a possible out during their darkest moments.

I did not find a woman who had attempted to end her life and would talk about it.

Perhaps this is because many people see suicide as the ultimate failure to cope, the ultimate weakness of self and of spirit. Yet others see it as the right choice, for some who know their quality of life is only going to get worse and have access to assisted dying.

Sherry, a counsellor at a women's crisis centre,

recommends unburdening grief and anger on paper.

"I have always written my way out of hell. I think, before cancer, I suspected that I wasn't really the woman I pretended to be. Looking back over this experience thus far, I see that I am precisely her. That's in the journal.

"In ways, I am safer in myself than I have ever been. I have always suspected that I was alone and have always befriended myself on paper. Thank God for that knowledge! It brought me through this from the beginning. Sometimes, I am sure that the only thing my sanity depends on is a pen with which I am comfortable!"

Keeping a journal can give you a way to begin to sort out your feelings. It can work as catharsis, writing out unexpressed anger, sadness, guilt, joy, fears, sexual fantasies.

Your journal is a place where every emotion is allowed, where you can be honest and be safe, where you can discover new insights and strengths.

It also allows you to look back and see that you are making progress on your journey.

"Some days I know my cancer was caused by the nine months of over-the-counter diet pills I took. Other days I am sure it is pollution-related. And sometimes I think it is because I was a bad, bad girl. I had an abortion…" Sherry wrote.

This is guilt. Like depression, guilt is anger that is turned within. "My husband hates me for this guilt," Sherry wrote.

But does he? She hadn't asked him.

"Bobby is young and healthy. I was a departure for him from the start. Freaked out, frizzy-haired, running from a weird marriage. He was so young, so normal, and here I come writhing through primal therapy, sometimes brilliant, more often idiotic, with my strange psychic shit, bizarre history, crazy family, and now this. But this is serious."

Sherry felt guilty about a lot of things.

She was, she thought, too emotional, too individualistic, too "different." Having cancer was just one more thing "wrong" with her in her husband's eyes, she thought. One more way she'd failed him and their marriage.

Several women said they believe their cancer has "hurt" their families, and added that they try to "act well" to make up for the damage they believe they've done to the people around them.

"I feel responsible for my illness," Donna wrote. "I succumbed to cancer. It was my weakness. Now, I have decided to be strong and any disease wishing to relieve me of some other part of my body is going to have one hell of a fight on its hands!"

At some point, the anger turned inward is redirected.

Women get mad, as Donna did.

They resolve to fight the cancer. In the process, they may also vent their anger upon caregivers, particularly doctors, their families, their friends and their children and mates.

There is no cancer personality, but there is a survivor personality. It can be, and at times needs to be, a feisty one.

Cancer patients are notoriously difficult to please, doctors and nurses have told me.

We are, these caregivers say, an angry and demanding group.

We demand care and attention.

We're often uncooperative, not conforming to the docile customers doctors would prefer to treat.

We ask questions. We demand answers when, often, doctors have no answers to give. Or better treatments to offer.

We complain.

These same caregivers might be less critical if, as a

part of their training, they had to endure a week of having a major illness, or even a week of being treated as if they had a major illness.

It could be quite eye-opening for them. Perhaps they'd gain some empathy.

This display of emotions by people with cancer is not only healthy, it may even contribute to our survival.

A Johns Hopkins study published in *The Journal of the American Medical Association* concluded that long term survivors of breast cancer are more likely to show the emotions of grieving, while deniers are less likely to survive.

The anger women feel was reflected in what they told me.

Sherry, who wrote out her pain and confusion, also wrote out her anger: "It was an anger so real, so white, of such force! It frightened me. I had never felt such anger before."

One evening, she pounded a table so hard that she bruised her hand and shattered the table. That lashing out shocked her. She had never acted so violently. The episode of the table trashing, she said, makes her wonder now if she wasn't being a bit dramatic. But at the time, her fury was very real. And, having expressed it, she felt purged.

Instead of working out her anger, as Sherry did, Barbara chose to swallow it. Her lover could not face her, literally, after she lost her breast to cancer.

He was a weak man who deserted her.

"The anger was the stage that lasted the longest," she wrote. "I was really pissed off, especially at that bastard!"

Women feel betrayed by mates who deny that there is a major problem.

"Just go get the operation and get it over with," Sally's husband said. Like it was an appointment for a haircut. She was angry, and who could blame her?

Other offenders targeted for wrath: family members who patronize and pamper but will not listen.

Doctors, particularly when a diagnosis or sign of recurrence is missed, or when they will not honestly answer a woman's questions, or when they try to sugar-coat bad news or when they are arrogant and condescending. Or dismissive.

Friends or family members who vanish when they are most needed.

Counsellors who mouth jargon and hide behind medical terminology.

Co-workers, who shun or are overly solicitous.

Employers afraid to hire or re-hire or who shuffle an employee off to do 'less taxing' work; in effect, a demotion.

Insurance companies whose premiums double or triple or suddenly cancel coverage.

Worse than the anger, many women said, were the fears. The first of these and the greatest is the fear of dying. "Accepting the fact that I might die" was the greatest hurdle for Jan, whose mother had died of breast cancer when she was 55.

On the back of the questionnaire, Jan listed the family members who had cancer: her mother, an uncle, a cousin, her sister, herself.

"It's in my family," she wrote. Of the five who had cancer, three have died. Cancer, to Jan, means death. This is a fear she cannot shake, even though she and her sister have survived.

Barbara also told of a history of cancer on both sides of her family. "I felt it was the kiss of death when I learned I had cancer," she wrote. "I had a very negative impression of cancer, because my mother died of it [when she was a child in the 1950s, when] radiation therapy was just beginning and Mother didn't respond to radiation. So, I felt there was no hope, in any way, for anyone who contracted cancer."

We must all come to grips with the fear of our own death, psychologists point out.

But most of us can shove that fear to a rear corner of our minds (psychoanalyst Dr. Jay Lefer calls this positive denial) along with other fears so that we can continue to function.

"In the most basic sense, you can't go around thinking, 'I'm going to die' even though it's an indisputable fact that we all will eventually," Dr. Lefer points out. The key word, of course, is "eventually."

To most of us, eventually is relegated to the murky future, when we are very old, when we have seen our children and even our grandchildren grow up, when we have had many years to do what we set out to do with our lives.

When we have lived fully, for a very long and healthy time.

The fear of death is tied in with the fear of not accomplishing goals, not living to see children well launched in the world, never meeting our grandchildren.

It's the fear, also, of other losses: your mate or lover, job and status. It's the fear of deformity, recurrence, helplessness, pain.

When she had cancer Lynn, who is 39, felt that she'd sailed through her cancer survival. After surgery and recovery, she worked part-time as a secretary while also taking a course to become a medical technologist and, with her husband, raising their two sons.

She barely had enough hours in the day, she thought, and didn't have the time to become involved in the cancer support group offered by her Minnesota cancer centre.

"My family was great, so were my friends. I was just too busy! I didn't need any other help!" she recalls.

But that changed a year ago when Lynn learned the cancer had returned.

"It hits you harder, the second time," she said. "After the first time, each anniversary was something to celebrate, on the way to that five-year mark [cancer-free, the medical definition of "cure."] I only made it to two. That was a real disappointment!"

We want so much to believe that the worst is past.

We tend to see the return of cancer not only as a setback in our health, but as a failure within ourselves, a failure to resist illness and a failure of the will to heal.

But it is the nature of cancer, and of diabetes and multiple sclerosis and some other health conditions, to become chronic. There is no cure.

After Lynn's recurrence, she made time for a support group, because she realized she needed to reach out for support and help in learning to accept that cancer is ongoing.

To come to accept this, you must search for a balance, between being overly cautious and watchful for recurrence, which can lead to obsessive concern on the one hand, or fatalistic disregard for your health on the other.

You must find a balance between hope and self-delusion, and between realistic expectation and despair.

To be able to do this, you must come to know the healthy woman who lives within your less-than-perfect body.

The fear of further losses, of recurrence or early death are real, rational fears for people with cancer.

When these fears did become fact, most women reached within to find ways to cope.

They found another job, another mate or lover.

They did what they could to minimize deformity, to develop new strengths, to find new interests and friends. For some, cancer did recur and treatment was repeated.

Many had periods of helplessness and loneliness and

pain. When these feared losses did happen, most women found that their efforts to recoup or come to accept what could not be changed were less difficult than they had imagined in darker moments. For most, the fear was worse than the reality.

The fears of death, further loss, or of deformity are all rational fears because any of these things can happen after cancer. There are also the irrational fears, things that probably won't happen but which we agonize over, sometimes endlessly.

After my mastectomy, I worried that my sisters would develop breast cancer, because I'd had it.

I also developed an exaggerated fear of being raped. This was more than taking the usual sensible self-protective precautions every woman takes to avoid assault. I became obsessed with the belief that I must safeguard myself from being raped, not because it would be another traumatic event further complicating my recovery, but because I had convinced myself that if I were ever raped the rapist would surely kill me. He would see that I was deformed, I imagined, and in his anger at being cheated, of accidentally assaulting a damaged body, he would stab me to death.

This nightmare played over and over in my mind until I was afraid of going out in the evening, afraid always that I had forgotten to lock my doors, afraid of being followed -- and all this when I lived in a small, friendly town with one of the lowest assault rates on the continent!

Imagine, feeling sorry for a potential rapist because he would be short-changed by a victim who appeared, when dressed, to be a normal woman with breasts intact!

This is a completely irrational fear, but I found other women who had a mastectomy or hysterectomy and share this same rape fear and 'feeling sorry' for the potential rapist!

Taking such crazy fears and examining them under the light of reason is very difficult to do when you have been rendered so psychologically and emotionally vulnerable.

It is something like telling yourself that you are just having a dream while you are still asleep and in the midst of a particularly grisly nightmare.

It can be very hard to wake yourself up.

This is one more area where an understanding listener, whether a friend or a counsellor, can help you see these fears for what they really are, irrational fantasies.

Once you see these fears clearly, and can talk about

why they have had you in their grip (for example, the poor rapist fear was based on self pity and low self esteem, as in "Not even a rapist could stand to see me now") you can begin to let these fears go.

Along the way, it can be hard to believe that your mourning will ever come to an end, yet, near the end of mourning, there does come a resolution to loss called acceptance. There comes a time when you can also let go of your depression, anger and guilt.

"I want my life back, but the thought of scrambling and rushing towards goals seems almost absurd," Sherry wrote just a few months after her mastectomy, as she shuttled between depression, anger, self-pity and guilt.

At that time, acceptance seemed unattainable, impossible: "I have always been such a clumsy, haphazard person. Now, I want to be fooled. I want to stagger out the other side. I want all the old stuff to excite me again. Gifts don't do it. Stationery stores, clothes, music don't do it now. What is acceptance? I think it's coming, though I'm getting set to fight it. I must decide just what acceptance means. Does it mean I have to really integrate this shit? Does it mean I have to pretend that it didn't happen?"

No. Acceptance isn't denial.

It isn't "Well, let's just forget this all happened, shall

we?"

It isn't putting on a cheery face or being able to make jokes about the missing body part (like some cheesy stand-up comedienne).

Acceptance also isn't forgetting the pain or the changes cancer brings.

Rather, it's coming to a point where you believe that having had cancer is a part of your life, not all of your life; one of the experiences that has shaped you; made you the strong woman you are today.

Now, after cancer, it is very possible to meet former goals or create new ones, to plan, to dream, to enjoy your survival.

To enjoy your life.

Acceptance is coming out of the wilderness and back into the light. It is coming to terms with reality, and going on from there. It is, essentially, peace.

And freedom.

"After the initial reaction, how did you feel?" I asked women, hoping for insights into how we grieve the losses of cancer.

"Do you agree with psychiatrist Elizabeth Kubler-Ross that people facing death go through stages of grief? Dr. Kubler-Ross also wrote that the stages aren't necessarily in any order, and not everyone goes through every stage. Did you go through stages of grieving?"

The fervour of the replies surprised me.

Half denied completely that they had grieved, usually explaining why they rejected the whole concept of grieving, and sometimes in these answers, revealing that they had, indeed, grieved but could not talk about it.

Phyllis, a professor at a prestigious Eastern university and a prize-winning author, does not see grief in terms of stages. "I do not agree with any generalizations about cancer," she wrote. "In fact, they make me very angry. Each person has to cope in her own way."

But exactly half the women asked this question said that yes, they believe they grieved and that grieving does have stages.

Most also agree with Phyllis' belief that we each cope in our own way.

"I think I have experienced all the Kubler-Ross stages except bargaining," another woman wrote. "However, maybe my bargain is 'since my life has been spared up until now, I will learn to cope graciously.' It is possible that that has become my MO.

"I have been through the other stages more than once, and in no particular order. How gracious I have been is debatable. But I have tried to involve others in my psychological survival techniques."

Many women found that grieving, and coping, seems to be a continual cycle, gradually spiralling them back to grief, anger, depression and helplessness in turn until each is finally resolved.

Linda was 28 when she was told she had Hodgkin's Stage IV. That meant she could not survive for very long but miraculously, she has.

She wrote: "Sometimes it feels like I'm going through these stages one at a time, sometimes I can recognize when I'm in the middle of two or more at once, and sometimes they overlap. But, most importantly, I've learned that just because you have visited one stage doesn't mean that you'll never visit it again.

"For a long time, I thought that acceptance would come when I had realized or resolved my own death. Now, I see that acceptance is a part of living, like denial. It's daily."

Sherry agrees. "Sometimes I'm sure I'm past it. Then I get knocked over again by a dream or an incident that just highlights the difference, the complete change in my life, my views, all my perceptions.

"Acceptance is like a daily potential, but the stages,

all of them, play over and over again. I seem to go through complete cycles, through each healing level."

One woman thought she could, and really should, avoid mourning.

She saw it as self-pity.

In the end, she only managed to postpone her grief.

Donna wrote: "I had two mastectomies, the first one when I was 29, the second a year later. Before I had cancer, my breasts were a part of me I enjoyed having. I wish I could have them back. I fed two babies with my breasts. I derived intense sexual pleasure from them.

"I knew from the moment that I first suspected that I had cancer that self-pity was a pitfall to be avoided at all costs. So, I never allowed myself to feel sorry for myself. Oh, there would be the odd moment when I would feel deep regret, but I made sure those moments didn't drag on. That's what got me through the first year and a half and my two operations.

"Sometime during the third year, I realized there was something wrong with me emotionally. I was deeply depressed and for a long time I couldn't put a name to what was bothering me. Eventually, after much soul-searching and thought, I realized that I had never let myself grieve for the loss of my breasts. I had lost and buried them and never shed a tear or faced up to the fact that the situation was absolutely permanent.

"I had been so glad to still be alive that I hadn't realized that one could be glad to be alive and sad at the same time. At that time, I allowed myself to experience fully the sorrow I had denied, and after some time of grieving, I eventually came to feel better about the situation."

The self and the soul heal slowly.

The journey through the valley of grief can take several months, or sometimes several years.

Even after grief is resolved and acceptance gained, there are times of remorse, fears, guilt, sadness.

But these episodes become less intense, less wrenching, less difficult to overcome, because you've travelled these paths before. Now, you know the terrain. And you know your way back to the light.

As Donna said, we can each become "more accepting every day."

FIVE

Woman, Redefined

On a hot July afternoon, six women hiked high in the foothills of the Rockies. They trudged along a path twisting between slabs of rock, coming finally to the clearing where they would camp for the night.

The clearing sloped away to more rock and beyond the rock, they found that the stream they'd been following widened into a small pool.

With a whoop of delight, the women slipped off their packs and in a few moments, five of them had stripped and plunged in. The sixth sat on the rocks, dangling her feet in the icy water.

"Per," one woman called, "aren't you coming in?"

"Soon," Per replied, watching them splash and laugh.

"Oh, come on, it's great once you're in!"

Per hesitated. She could swim in her underwear, she thought, but she'd feel silly doing that, as if she were a prude. She watched one woman dive off a rock. Another had come out of the water and now lay naked in the sun.

They look so relaxed, Per thought wistfully. So free. She longed to feel the cool water on her tired, sweaty body, but... no. Her friends knew she'd had a mastectomy, but knowing is different than seeing. How would they react? What would they say?

She looked towards the campsite above, thinking perhaps she should start gathering firewood. Then she turned back to the water, and, on impulse, peeled off her shorts and blouse, panties and finally her bra. Arms folded protectively over the railroad scar where her left breast had been, she ran into the water.

Later, she laid on her stomach, the sun warming her skin, feeling strong and alive. As the six women sunned themselves and rested, they began to talk, about the day's hike, about what awaited them after returning home the next day, about themselves.

Feeling brave, Per asked her companions how they felt about seeing her changed body.

Their answers were honest but kind.

"They said loving, reassuring things. Some were also very curious, but no one was repulsed. One woman expected that I'd have some awful open wound. She was surprised by my nice smooth scar. No one jumped up to embrace me, but then, no one ran screaming from the mountain either."

For Per that moment of acceptance by other women at a mountain campsite marked her turning point towards accepting and making peace with her changed body and her changed self.

On that day, she says, she could finally say "this is the way my body is now."

Finally, she could stop apologizing for it, stop protecting other people.

At the moment that she undressed, it seemed to her that it was on impulse, but now she believes that this revelation of body and self was something she was finally ready to do. It had more to do with confidence in herself than in her body, Per said. It was not until afterward that she realized she'd been very nervous.

And it was liberating, she said. It simply isn't possible to feel confident and fully alive if you also feel that you must hide your body, or your feelings.

If you were to have an experience like Per's, perhaps while with a group of women at the lake together, relaxing and the talk turned to our most private feelings about our bodies, you would probably discover that every woman there over age 18 feels in some way deformed, or at least different.

I had that experience, too, at a friend's cottage, and I discovered:

- there is the one with the beautiful legs, who says she hates her body because she has "no waist."

- there is another very attractive woman, convinced she is fat because of her gently-rounded stomach

- and the one who had breast reduction surgery fifteen years ago. She is petite and lovely, but in her mind, she is still the unhappy teenager who was teased about her too-large breasts.

- and there is you.

It's sad, isn't it? Every woman has at least one feature that is attractive as well as some that are less than lovely but not anything near repulsive.

But most women ignore the positive and turn the somewhat average into, in their own view, something grotesque.

Besides creating a lot of needless unhappiness, this reverse vanity takes a tremendous amount of energy.

For a long time, I could see the truth in this -- for other women. I, on the other hand, had a right, I thought, to my anguish over my body because it truly was grotesque.

My two reconstructed breasts were like two oranges glued to my front. One was much larger than the other. They didn't look like my real breasts. They didn't feel like the originals either.

I had my natural breasts for just fifteen years, from the time they developed until they were lost due to cancer.

I plan on a long survival, so, in the entire expanse of my life, fifteen years will be only an interlude.

I will spend most of my life without my first breasts, but with reconstructed breasts. When I realised this, I stopped calling them, with bitter humour, my "fabulous fakes" and started calling them simply my breasts.

Not matched, not soft and warm and responsive to touch and not able to feed a baby.

But also, not flat or drooping.

And not possibly harbouring cancer.

Just mine.

You may have a reconstructed breast or vagina, or a

prosthetic arm, or a stoma. You may have difficulty accepting this change in your body; may even believe it is impossible to accept it.

But consider. Didn't you accept eye makeup, and possibly glasses or contacts, filled or capped teeth and a watch? And didn't all these attachments eventually feel like a part of you?

That is because these additions helped you see better, look better, chew your food without pain and get to work and appointments on time. Your cane or prosthesis or appliance also functions for you. If you cannot see it as attractive, can you appreciate it for the way it works for you?

Can you accept the changed part of your body as perhaps not your most alluring feature but among your average okay body parts? With the proviso that many of these prostheses and reconstructions weren't available until recently?

Today they are constantly being improved, so there is always the hope that you have better, more lifelike, and even more functional reconstruction or prostheses in the future.

For now, take advantage of the physical comforts that are available. During treatment, there are physical changes, most of them uncomfortable and all of them requiring adjustment. Since all of us react differently to treatment, and treatments are tailored to your type and stage of cancer, you should note these discomforts and ask your doctor to recommend or prescribe medications or other strategies you can use to feel better and to cope. If she doesn't know, keep looking. Someone has come this way before.

During chemotherapy, your sense of smell may become acute (making formerly pleasant odours, such as dinner cooking, overpowering and nauseating) and your sense of taste may also change. A craving for bread and other carbohydrates and inability to eat meat is another common reaction. If preparing food that you can't eat makes you sick, look for some alternatives. It may be that lighter fare (fresh salads, fish, fruit) is more appealing as well as easier to prepare.

Another member of the family can cook, while you go for a walk or rest in another part of the house. The people around you expect you to tell them how they can help you.

Do it.

Ask for what you need, if not for yourself, for them, because the people who love you want and need the opportunity to help you.

If you are undergoing chemotherapy, you will probably lose your hair. This usually happens just after your second chemotherapy treatment.

If you are going to lose your hair, it will come out not gradually but in handfuls, usually just leaving a few strands here and there.

Sometimes, you don't lose your hair but it becomes thin, dull and possibly turns darker in colour.

Either way, a wig can help you look and feel better.

If the cost is a hardship, some medical insurance and cancer support groups can help.

It's best to buy a wig before you start to lose your hair.

Try it on. Take a friend to help choose the most flattering style. Don't ask someone else to go and buy it for you, because fit is important.

More tips on choosing a wig:

- a real-hair wig is the best choice, because the synthetic ones are hotter, can cause your scalp to itch and they look less authentic.

- to hold it securely in place, use beautician's tape at the crown and the temple (ask your hairdresser to show you how to do this) and have it styled to suit you.

- if your wig is your usual hair colour and style, you can start wearing it before you begin to lose your hair.

- wash your wig once a week using shampoo.

Another aid that will help you feel better and sleep better is learning relaxation techniques and using them. There are many good books on this subject (ask your librarian or look at a bookstore or online) and many community colleges also offer courses in stress reduction. Using these techniques can ease side effects such as headaches and nausea and help you face your next treatment or doctor's appointment. Reducing stress will also strengthen your immune system and may ultimately help you survive.

After the end of treatment, your body will gradually begin to feel like home again. The peculiar side effects don't stop immediately. Some seem to fade away very gradually.

For example, a metallic mouth taste after radiation to your head or neck may linger for many months. With time the side effects go, and with them the fatigue. As your body begins to feel right and smell right once again, depression lifts. Periods become regular again, unless you no longer have a uterus and ovaries.

If you lost your hair, it grows back and is often thicker and curlier than it was before and may be a different colour.

While many of the side effects are gone by several months after treatment ends, some are permanent. Now, you must change what can be changed and come to accept what can't be changed.

What can be changed? Scars, for one thing. These can be surgically neatened.

A wide scar can be pulled tighter, for example.

For scars that cannot be improved, there are cosmetic concealers available at drug stores. While applying Vitamin E oil or aloe cream may improve the softness and appearance of scars, it usually can't eliminate them.

With time, they will fade and become less prominent.

Only a decade ago, breast reconstruction was still considered cosmetic surgery, but that is no longer true. It is replacement of a lost body part with a man-made facsimile, and the cost is usually covered, or at least partly-covered, by health insurance.

Some surgeons will do a reconstruction at the same time they do the mastectomy, which seems to me the most humane way, but others will not do reconstruction until after chemotherapy or radiation are completed. If you plan to have reconstruction, your surgeon and your plastic surgeon should examine you before the mastectomy. This allows both to do the best possible job for you in getting rid of the cancer and in leaving you with as little damage as possible.

Breast reconstruction may delay but will not prevent detection of a recurrence of cancer on the chest wall.

When I asked women how they felt about their reconstructed breasts, most were content with the result:

"My life has changed because I had reconstruction. I feel attractive again. I can wear my clothes and never worry about something slipping around," said Sharon, who is 39. "I like myself now and I'm very happy about the way I look."

"While it is quite well done, there is an imbalance. It's not perfect," Barbara wrote.

"After I had the mastectomy, there was no question about it: I hated myself. I hated to undress. If I really wanted to punish myself I would just stand and look in the mirror," Elena wrote. "I had no relationship with a man, so the only person I had to please was myself. I wasn't pleased. I'd buy clothing, and anything that I put on would never please me. It would always show. To me it showed.

"Other people, my daughter, would say 'It's okay. It doesn't show' but to me it always showed. Then a new type of prosthesis came out, a very expensive one that was supposed to stay close to your body, but it slipped around, and it was supposed to be warm, but it didn't do that either. It was just never right.

"I think for some people, these things aren't a problem, but for me it was. Probably all in my mind. But it was seven years before I got my reconstruction."

"I'd read about it. At the time, they wouldn't even talk about reconstruction for my type of mastectomy; they said there wasn't enough skin left to do it. So, it just never occurred to me to ask, because there wasn't anything there to work with.

"And I was so afraid. I was 53 years old, and it had been seven years since I had the mastectomy and I hadn't had a recurrence. One doctor said that it would start the cancer up again to have reconstruction. [false and another reason to always get a second opinion.]

"I was afraid of surgery again, of being weak, of how I'd be able to keep the house going, and my job, and maybe being disabled, afraid that the reconstruction wouldn't look right, and I had heard of women who have had it done and it doesn't work.

"It was a very difficult thing to do, just voluntarily present myself again at the hospital, but I did it, and it's good. I had a breast made [from a flap of skin taken from elsewhere on your body – belly, back or thighs]. I'm satisfied with the way it is. I'm able to wear the clothes that I want, and do everything I want to do. It pleases me.

"I did have some depression after the reconstruction, while my body was hurting. And then as soon as I didn't have the pain anymore, the depression went away. Not overnight. Gradually.

"Sure, the reconstruction doesn't look the way it did [her natural breast did] and another person might look at my new breast and say 'Yech! That's awful!' but I look at it and I think it is very good.

"I feel better about myself than I ever have in my life. I feel good when I look at myself. I feel normal again. It's like I was given a second chance to be happy."

Some women who don't have cancer choose to have a mastectomy. These are women who are at high risk or afraid who are very much afraid they may eventually develop cancer. Angelina Jolie, the actress, is one woman who made this choice for this reason.

This surgery, called prophylactic mastectomy, has always been controversial. Opponents point out that it is wrong to cut off a body part that is totally healthy, just because it may some day become ill.

They add that with careful breast self-examination and regular blood tests and scans, breast cancer can be caught early.

On the other side, surgeons who do prophylactic mastectomies say that they provide peace of mind. Some plastic surgeons believe they can achieve better results if both breasts are reconstructed at the same time.

My own second mastectomy, performed at the time of breast reconstruction, was prophylactic. My surgeon said he could not offer "a good match" after reconstruction unless both breasts were reconstructed and I allowed myself to be swayed to his belief. Now, I regret sacrificing my healthy left breast. My reconstructed breasts did not match. One was larger and lower on my chest than the other.

My first reconstruction was in 1980; methods and results have improved very much since then. And there is another danger: the choice of implants. I had a silicone breast implant (since recalled and no longer used) that broke, allowing silicone to spread through my body. Getting it right – saline implants – gave me a better result, but it required three surgeries to get there.

If I had it to do again, I would not trade a healthy, functioning breast just to try to achieve what a surgeon calls "a better match."

It is a lasting regret. I could have breastfed our son if I had resisted that surgeon's coercion to agree to something that only made the job easier for him.

There was a time when I rejected prophylactic mastectomy for any woman, seeing it as mutilation as pointless and cruel as removing young women's clitorises to prevent them from masturbating, a common practice still in some cultures.

Now, I believe prophylactic mastectomy may be justified for psychologic, but never for merely cosmetic, reasons. Let me give an example.

A friend's elderly mother is terrified of developing breast cancer.

She has seven sisters, and of the seven, five have had cancer and three have died after having cancer. Each morning for over thirty years my friend's mother has woken with the belief that this will be the day she finds the lump in her breast.

"Breast cancer absolutely terrifies her!" my friend says. "Cancer [fear] has destroyed her life!" For this woman, a mastectomy performed years ago could have saved her having to live in this hell of fear.

My friend agrees. There are people for whom the fear of cancer is considerably worse than the treatment for it.

For these women, I believe, prophylactic mastectomy or hysterectomy (if they fear uterine cancer) could be the wisest choice.

Women who do not choose breast reconstruction (and each woman must decide this for herself) have the option of wearing a breast prosthesis. These can be as simple as a foam or cloth pad, ranging up to a custom made, flesh-colored silicone jell-filled prosthesis.

Most health insurance plans cover the cost.

If you choose to wear a prosthesis, buy the very best one you can afford and have it fitted.

A good, weighted prosthesis will fill in any hollows under your arm left by surgery, look and feel natural under clothing and next to your skin, and the good ones are comfortable, women who wear them say.

There are three potential problems with a breast prosthesis: it may slip out of place (but a carefully-fitted prosthesis - fitted in a mastectomy bra or clothing with a mastectomy pocket shouldn't); if punctured, they will leak (so would a breast implant), and, unlike a reconstructed breast, a breast prosthesis does not have a nipple.

If your cancer was of the jaw or head, skin and bone grafts can rebuild your face, along with prostheses. For most people with cancer of the jaw or face, dental reconstruction is necessary.

A combination of plastic surgery and prostheses can make it possible to speak and eat again. These new face and neck parts look very real. Skin is colored to match your own and can even have freckles. It is also easily cleaned and durable.

Beth, a nurse who lost her vagina when she was 22, chose a reconstructed vagina despite being warned of the disadvantages, which include needing to learn how to use a new vagina.

She wrote: "The first attempt at intercourse was a mess. Orgasm was nowhere for me. Tears and tears could not express my feelings of this added loss. I thought I may as well be dead."

But she persevered, seeing a social worker and looking for innovative ways to be sexual.

"My new grafted vagina served a utilitarian purpose, since there was no feeling or sensation except that of fullness or penetration. I found I had to give [my lover] directions to what areas were sensitive and arousable. My nerve sensation around my labia and clitoris was less than 50 per cent of what it had been. Touching, caressing, and experimenting -- I could be orgasmic in new ways, such as through breast and neck stimulation and fantasy. These orgasms were different, but sexually satisfying."

It took Beth over two years to accept her changed

body and her changed self, and, as she explained, it took a lot of work and a lot of faith and courage. And patience. In the process, she renewed more than her own sexual self. She restructured her life.

Acceptance and renewal, the woman you are after cancer and beyond cancer, requires separating your self from the cancer. You are not the cancer, and you are not the scars it has left.

It was merely a disease, that you had.

Acceptance also means assimilating the cancer experience, and your changed body, into a working definition of who you are today.

It is a shift in attitude, from victim to survivor to cancer veteran to fully alive woman. "I am a beautiful woman with a great job, two nice kids, a loving man, and incidentally, one breast" is very different from "I'm damaged. I have a great job, nice kids, a supportive lover, but those don't matter. They don't help. I am reduced, as a woman and as a person. I am a non-person."

When I asked what renewal meant, Marti, who doesn't have a job and is raising her kids alone on Mother's Allowance, gave a simple and moving answer: "It is a renewal of my love for myself, with a greater amount of self respect."

Other women added that it meant greater freedom

from self-consciousness, freedom to feel good again.

It meant increased patience with oneself and tolerance and compassion for others. I asked women how they came to this state of renewal. Here is their advice:

Take care of yourself

Eating properly, for instance, is much more difficult if you are still having chemotherapy or radiation treatments or if you live alone, but make the effort. What you eat has a direct effect on how you feel.

If you can't eat healthily, at least take vitamin supplements. Get enough rest and daily exercise.

Exercise is helpful for three reasons: first, being fit is something you can achieve. It won't give you back your 18-year-old body, but it will certainly give you a body that looks and feels better.

The second reason is that exercise gets your adrenalin pumping and so helps your immune system.

Exercise is also an effective anti-depressant, creating a natural high.

Other helpers women recommended: hypnosis, biofeedback, acupuncture, massage, yoga, affirmations, meditation, mindfulness, travel, hobbies, playing with pets.

Ask for help, and, when you ask, be specific

When your fridge is empty but you've just had a chemotherapy treatment and you don't have the strength to shop, phone a friend and ask her to do that chore.

If you can't ask for specific chores (I need you to invite my kids for a sleepover; cut the grass, take my car for an oil change, come over and just be a friend for an hour) appoint a friend to field offers of help. Then, when people say something like, "let me know if you need help," you can say, "Of course. Susan is looking after this for me. Here's her number."

Make a list of your questions and concerns, and take it to your next appointment with your doctor. If she can't answer in a way that is comprehensible, ask her to refer you to someone who can help you with the information you need.

Forget the strong soldier stance and take advantage of all the help you can get. Now's the time to call in your markers, because no one should have to get through this without help!

"Cry"

Allow yourself to grieve.

When she tried to skip grieving, Donna sunk so deeply into depression that she considered suicide.

The shock of realizing she might die, not because of the cancer but because of her deep depression, forced her to examine her life.

"Cancer made me decide, finally, to live. I asked myself, 'What do you want to do, Donna?' and the answer was "LIVE!'"

After a crisis, it is natural to confront the tough questions: Who am I? Where is my life going? What do I really want? It helps to remind yourself of the person you are, aside from being a woman with cancer, as in "I am an active woman who loves camping and hiking, I am a creative woman who enjoys entertaining, I am a caring woman . . . and if I start doing these things I enjoy again, I will feel like my regular self again."

Know exactly why you want to live

To reach an important goal, to realize a dream, to build a good relationship with someone you cherish, to have a child, to raise the children you have and launch them into adulthood…know your reasons why your life matters and why it is worth saving.

Choose activities you enjoy

For Mildred, who wrote to me after she happened to see an article I had written about surviving cancer in *The Toronto Star* while she was visiting family in Ontario, it is music that makes life meaningful. After returning home to England, she wrote:

"I was hustled in for a mastectomy 16 years ago. I conduct choirs, so it was an immediate challenge to raise, fully-extend and wave around my right arm, if I did not want to relinquish my leadership. As soon as the worst of the effects of the deep-ray treatment [radiation] had healed over, I took a forward look to what oratorio we were going to do next!"

For her 71st birthday gift while in Canada, Mildred and her family went to an amusement park where she "rode on all the thrilling water shoots, chair-o-planes, roller coasters" and had "a glorious time."

Back in Manchester, Mildred wrote that she was now "hearing how the music has progressed during our absence. My choirs help me raise money for cancer research, hoping that others may lead a full and happy life, as I am privileged to do!"

Several women told of learning new leisure activities.

Others wrote to say they had gone back to school, at age 40 or 50 and beyond, so they could pursue a career they'd always dreamed of having.

Work, whether it is paid or unpaid, is important, sociologists say. It provides self esteem builders such as recognition, acceptance and accomplishment. It puts us in touch with other people we might not ever meet otherwise, and it gives order and stability to our lives.

Sigmund Freud put it well when he said that work "is man's strongest tie to reality."

Of course, not all jobs are so rewarding.

If you have a job that makes you unhappy, re-examine your reasons for staying. You may find these reasons no longer seem as important as they once did.

Barbara, who is 48, had this experience: "I quit my job and returned to school, majoring in social work, an area in which I feel I can help others. I am particularly interested in working with women and I'm becoming more and more interested in working with the elderly. I also want to travel and live in Europe for at least a year.

"How can I afford this; you ask? Well, I have new priorities and goals. I'm using the money I got from my divorce, which I had salted away for my old age."

"I'm more interested in living in the here and now, and let the future take care of itself, which it will!"

Give yourself at least one good laugh a day

In **Anatomy of an Illness**, Norman Cousins relates how he survived a life-threatening disease by checking himself out of hospital, into a hotel, and taking control of his own cure.

A large part of that cure involved watching funny movies, and, Cousins wrote, "It worked. I made the joyous discovery that ten minutes of genuine belly laughter had an anaesthetic effect and would give me at least two hours of pain-free sleep."

Many women said keeping their sense of humour was central to their healing. Any humour, even black humour, can relieve pain and help you cope.

Stop punishing yourself for what you're not

If you're feeling guilty, whatever your past 'sins' were, forgive yourself! How bad was whatever you did, anyway?

It wasn't as bad as murder, was it?

Even most murderers eventually get parole.

Set yourself free!

Give up the cultural myths!

Particularly the beauty myth, the perfection myth and the happily ever after myth. These are all impossible dreams.

Try this:

Give yourself an uninterrupted half hour alone. Put on some soft music, pour yourself some wine or make tea and use your favourite goblet or cup. Consciously let go of the day's concerns.

Then slowly undress. When you are nude, look at your body in a mirror. What do you see and who do you see reflected there? Probably what you will see first are things about your body that you are very critical of -- surgery scars, perhaps laugh lines, stretch marks from pregnancy, a tummy bulge.

What else?

What parts of your body can you admire? Name them.

Consider for a moment what would happen if you stopped classifying your body into these two lists of good and bad or acceptable and ugly parts.

Let us say that, just for a few moments, you see each part of your body the way you think of your eye colour. One colour isn't superior to any other. All babies are born with blue or brown eyes, and within days the colour their eyes will remain is set for life.

Blue isn't any prettier than brown, it just is. And we accept this without ever agonizing over it. It is the same with breasts, stomachs, hips, legs. One shape isn't necessarily any better than another. It is just the cultural hype that says it is.

Why believe this?

Take a closer look at your face.

Are there laugh lines?

Maybe small wrinkles?

And your body. With a finger, trace the scars or stomas left by surgery. Feel their sensitivity to touch. Notice how they are fading and healing.

Remember that you are looking at these scars without judging. They are not beautiful; they are not ugly.

They just are.

Look at your reflection and say aloud: "These are part of my body now. My body can never be perfect. But it can be healthy and strong, and I know there is beauty in strength.

"I have survived.

"I am strong.

"And I am a beautiful woman!"

Pour your wine or tea, because it is time for the toast. Looking into the mirror, lift your goblet, or cup, and say "I do have a mastectomy scar (or a neck scar, or a stoma) and I do have stretch marks and I do have a tummy (or full hips) and I do have great legs and attractive hands . . . and I don't look like a model or a movie star.

I look better than that!

Because all these things, the scars and all of it, are the

medals of honour I have earned in a life fully lived with a well-lived in body.

Ask a friend to help

If you can't quite believe this toast to yourself, after honestly trying it several times, ask a close friend to look at your body and tell you truthfully what she sees. Ask her to be specific.

Perhaps she will offer some suggestions on things you can change, such as trying a new hairstyle or makeup.

Chances are, those parts of your body you think of very negatively she will see as "not all that bad" or even "better than most of the women I've seen at the gym."

You might also ask your lover/mate what he/she thinks of your body -- all of it, including the changed parts.

Joy was surprised to discover that her lover, now her husband, found the loss of her pubic hair erotic. When he told her that, the loss of her hair caused by chemotherapy suddenly seemed less traumatic.

When you ask for a reaction from a friend or mate, you will probably hear that they value you for who you are.

While your mate may mourn the loss of your breast

or vagina or leg or nose, he or she also rejoices that you have survived. And if they truly love you, they love all of you, not just selected parts.

Anyone who says they can't love you after cancer didn't really love you before.

And you deserve better than that.

Be kind to yourself

Congratulate yourself. Show yourself the compassion you would show a loved one if it had been him or her who had gone through a similar life trauma or accident.

That means small indulgences like new cushions to brighten your living room or a weekend away and larger ones, like trying something you've always wanted to do, or moving to a place you've always wanted to live, or travel.

"My focus used to be on my man," Per wrote. "Now, it is on me, on my life!" Love the one you'll always be with -- you!

Expect your body to help you live well

Your body, after all, is a heroine as much as you are. You and your body have come this far together. Together you must make it worth all the hard work and pain of surviving. This may mean relearning to use your arm, to walk, to have an orgasm. If you need aids to live, such as prosthesis or catch bags, accept them as your life preservers.

Expect others to see the beauty in you

Think of yourself as beautiful and others will, too. But if you are constantly putting yourself down, you will give them no choice but to agree with you.

Have faith

This means faith in the religious sense, if that is a meaningful part of your life, but also faith in yourself, and in your ability to heal and renew yourself.

Nancy, who had breast cancer when she was 49, wrote, "For the first time in many years, I began to pray, just to have someone to talk to. My God is a Superior Being who is Father/Mother and the Mother aspect of my God has been very important to me at this time.

"I talked to Her in the car, while driving to treatments, waiting for treatments, X-rays, blood work. I used Mother/God as a focus to stay sane when I felt like my world was falling apart."

Faith also means being positive. Here's one way you can put this to work. Instead of fighting discomfort or pain, allow yourself to move with it. Don't fight it. Accept, with faith, while reminding yourself that you can get through it and that it will ease up with the pain control methods you have chosen. This faith in your body to go with the pain has two effects: it can lessen the pain while helping you relax. That preserves your strength and your immunity.

Live in the moment

"Watching my uncle die of cancer, I learned so much about living for the moment," Toni wrote. "Later, when I found I had cancer, too, I was ready. I knew I had to live for now."

Barbara left her lover and her job (both had been unsatisfactory for a long time) and went back to school, at 48. Cancer, she says, jolted her out of her complacent life, and into a new, more rewarding one.

"I really like myself so much better now," she wrote. "I'm a much more positive person. I feel extra strength because I not only survived, but I did it with grace and flair!"

For others following the path through cancer to acceptance and triumph, she offered this advice: "Don't despair! You are alive. Your life will have more meaning, and you will become stronger because of the cancer. Trust me! And trust yourself!"

Life is no rose garden and isn't meant to be. "There are still night moments of fear," Nancy wrote, "but I also feel closer to my mate, more intensely aware of each day, focused on my priorities and eager to live!"

Only you determine the joy you get from each day of your life.

INTIMACY

SIX – YOU AND YOUR MATE

SIX

You and Your Mate

"We have been married for 20 years, and I would call it a good marriage. When I had my first mastectomy, my husband was very gentle, very kind. He told me, 'I loved you before and I love you now. Nothing can change that!'

"But even though he said that, my feelings about my own femininity and my self were very low for a long time. Living through it made me strong.

"The bond between my husband and I is even closer." – Sharon, 39, who has had two mastectomies.

"Before, I didn't think much about my breasts, except that they were very small. My husband kept reinforcing that belief. Now he tells me that I'm ugly. He says he's doing me a favor when he uses me to relieve himself – that's what sex is with him. I allow him to do it. It's easier than having to play games. We've had a very unsatisfactory sex life throughout our 31 years of marriage." – Sally, 49, who had a mastectomy two years ago.

What happens to committed relationships after a woman has cancer? Do couples grow closer, or do they tend to be wrenched apart? And how can couples keep their relationships strong?

Caregivers often say, "If it was good before, it will be good again." This sounds simplistic but it holds a truth.

Cancer does not destroy marriages. Good marriages stay good or become even stronger, as Sharon's did.

Troubled relationships, like Sally's, generally get worse.

The middle majority of comfortable, stable, 'OK' marriages tend to be just as stable after cancer.

To put it another way, the relationship 'rich' get richer, the 'poor' get poorer, and the rest ultimately stay about the same. But in the time from the initial diagnosis, through treatment ups and downs and adjustment, when a woman is grieving her loss and when her mate is also grieving that loss, the cancer crisis does strain their relationship. Sometimes to the breaking point.

To speak of quality in relationships, we must start with a definition. What are the ingredients of a good marriage?

Counselors generally agree that a strong marriage is one of equals who are partners in creating a life of mutual respect, caring, affection and shared interests. In a good marriage, both partners feel they can express their true feelings and needs, knowing that their partner will meet these needs or support their mate in achieving their goals.

Among relational needs are companionship. Giving and receiving sexual pleasure is another.

Sally's husband didn't suddenly become an ogre in bed and everywhere else because she had breast cancer, but he did use cancer as an excuse to act even more miserably toward her.

Looking towards the opposite end of the relationship quality continuum, Sharon's husband treated her in a gentle and kind way because he has always been a kind and supportive mate. Mutual caring was the established pattern of their marriage.

While it is a qualified truth to say that after a period of crisis and emotional upheaval, relationships do return to their former texture and quality, it is untrue that crises such as cancer (or bankruptcy, or the loss of a child, or other major misfortunes) necessarily strengthen relationships.

It is truer to say that any crisis challenges the relationship just as it challenges the people who have formed that relationship. Couples with flimsy coping skills or with weak links to each other may get along until the going gets tough, then break under the pressures.

This is a common pattern and may explain why couples whose relationships appeared solid before cancer may separate after diagnosis according to John Lamont, a gynecologist and Professor of Obstetrics and Gynecology at McMaster University in Hamilton, Ontario.

Affairs (involving either mate) and separation or divorce do sometimes follow a cancer diagnosis, but it is too easy to see one spouse's cancer as the culprit. Before looking at how intimacy and its physical expression, sexuality, change after cancer, let's briefly consider how intimacy and sexuality function in long-term relationships before cancer.

Our culture strongly encourages women to be primarily relaters and men to be attainers. As children, we learn that these behaviors are expected of us. As adults, most women define themselves in terms of their relationships, their connectedness with other people. Most men tend to define themselves using an accomplishment scale that is outward looking – job title, earning power, occupying the corner office.

Even relationships are measured in an accomplishment context, as either successful or a failure, happy or miserable. For women, taught from early childhood to be relational, to nurture, to facilitate communication, relationship success (or failure) and happiness (or unhappiness) is defined differently.

While more women today recognize their own needs and desires for both career and personal attainment, this can lead to another set of false expectations, the Having It All syndrome. But despite career responsibilities and accomplishments, women still are expected (and we expect ourselves) to be the primary nurturers of the people in our lives, particularly our children, our mates and our own aging parents.

But because our lovers are predominantly male (except for the ten percent of women who choose female lovers) the love partner is likely to be someone who has learned, from an early age, to be uncomfortable expressing his needs, especially his emotional needs.

Although this is changing, men still tend to view

intimacy as vulnerability, a position men and many women abhor.

Intimacy means a man must share 'the truth' about his inner self, including his weak self and his fearful self. To need and to love, and admit it, is to risk humiliation and rejection.

Men (and some women) want to be close, but at the same time they are afraid of being unmasked – having to face emotions they have avoided ever thinking about.

To take off the protective armor is to risk being seen as soft, or worse, effeminate.

By avoiding intimacy, many men believe they can avoid emotional pain. Many women are just as afraid of rejection but women, as a group, are more emotionally brave. Not only are we social and relational, our brains are more verbal, more able to communicate than are male brains.

Women are more willing to take the risk, and to keep on taking it to find intimate fulfillment in relationships.

Men tend to prefer career risk, ambition risk, financial risk – but not relationship risk.

Our misconception, as women, is not in avoiding intimacy but in believing we can have it if we want it, while also having everything else we want, too. We would like to believe that we have the energy to simultaneously grab all the good things in life.

Men more realistically expect to put most of their energy and strength into their preferred areas of risk: career, etc.

While women may be bolder in exploring the inner worlds of intimacy, it is widely believed that men have a much clearer, much less conflicted view of their own sexuality.

To many women, sex is the proof of love. Therefore, if he has sex with me, he must love me. For us, the feelings of sensuality ("I need you," "I need to touch you," "I want to give you pleasure,") and the feelings of love are the same. As women we have a strong need to believe that sex = love.

To most men, sex = sex. Love is something else. This 'disconnect' probably had quite a lot to do with the survival of our species.

Women secretly yearn to be swept away on a flight of romantic fantasy with dreamlike lovers who somehow, magically, know how (and when and where) to lead them to ecstasy. [Of course, this sounds like the stuff of every romance novel. It never fails to entrance women readers who want to live, and re-live, this experience.]

Most men know exactly what their body needs to feel aroused and fulfilled and to them there is nothing magical about it. Men are less likely to use, or require, fantasy to reach orgasm with a partner (although men may use fantasy to masturbate).

But it is a myth, says psychologist Bernie Zilbergeld in **Male Sexuality** that men never suffer sexual self-doubt or confusion. Of course, they do. Some people of both genders fake interest, arousal and orgasms on occasion, but for different reasons. While a woman may fake it to avoid hurting her mate's feelings, men pretend to climax to portray their own sexual confidence.

And, says Dr. Zilbergeld, everyone believes the myth that everyone else is having lots and lots of great sex (much better than what you're having, or wish you were having). Although many men are (usually secretly) just as romantic as women, generally men are socialized to think of sex as straightforward and more physical than emotional. Just like sports.

Men have learned that sex is goal-oriented, and the goal is orgasm. So, to most men, the candlelit dinner for two, a gentle neck massage, a pat on the bum may be nice, but they aren't sex.

For men caught in this socially-induced sexual rut, sex is intercourse. Period. Foreplay, after play and sensual pleasuring may be pleasant enough or may merely be what you must do to get her in the mood.

Women need intimacy, or at least an aura of intimacy, to enjoy sex. For most men, sex without intimacy is OK. As Dr. Zilbergeld says, many men do not know how to be emotionally intimate. They don't know what they are missing, and they can't risk finding out.

Physically, men and women experience arousal in very similar ways, but we have learned to have very different requirements before we can allow our arousal to happen.

Women need to relax to be able to enjoy sex; men use sex to relax. For men, sex is an escape from worries and distractions. Most women must consciously relax and clear their minds of other concerns to allow arousal.

Try explaining to a man that the phone ringing or a baby in the next apartment crying or your teenagers still clumping around the house outside your closed door end the flow of delicious feelings for you, and how hard it is to get those feelings back.

Few men even hear these distractions when they are aroused.

For women (and some men) sexual arousal is the culmination of feelings throughout the day. Women carry all the anger, frustration or pleasure gathered from all their encounters that day, including with lovers.

Men, it is believed, are more capable of compartmentalizing any unpleasantness or worry, more easily clearing the way for arousal, even when they're tired. Therapists say the complaint, "You're always too tired!" is much more often made by husbands than by wives.

Men also can more easily become excited by visual triggers (tight jeans, garters, boots, you in nothing but one of his old shirts) than women can.

Consider tastes in erotica, and how they tend to divide by gender. Men generally favor photographs and movies of sex in progress, while women prefer stories about sexual relationships stressing the sensuality.

Here are two reflections of these tastes: men buy pictures of women looking alluring (*Playboy*) while women buy increasingly 'hot' or steamy/erotic romance novels (**50 Shades of Gray**).

Most women feel close to their lovers when they share their feelings, which means talking about these feelings. Men generally do not express their feelings or analyze them, and they especially do not talk about sexual feelings.

Women want to hear how men feel about them: "Why don't you ever say that you love me?" while men think that sex is communication, that it replaces communications somehow, as in "I don't have to say it; we're married." Or "Doesn't what we just did prove it?"

For women, emphasis is on the quality of intimacy, and if the sex is less than good, they will put up with it to keep the relationship. Many women prefer cuddling to intercourse, as agony aunt Ann Landers found in her famous survey in the '80s.

Pepper Schwartz has studied the sexual habits of heterosexual and homosexual Americans. She has found that when the sex is less than fulfilling, husbands are more likely than their wives to either have an affair or want to separate.

Dr. Schwartz also points out the difference between the genders when it comes to doing the sexual inviting.

Men, she says, feel inhibited about refusing sex, while women feel inhibited about asking for it.

Women tend to want their partners to know when they want sex, by some subtle signals. Partners are expected to know the code.

Many men wish their partners would be more active, more open, even occasionally aggressive in initiating sex, Dr. Schwartz says, but "men want their women to become tigresses in bed only up to a point and women are supposed to know where that point is.

If a couple can manage a kind of 50:50 refusal and initiation, they tend to be happier about their sex life and happier in their relationship," Dr. Schwartz concludes.

If it is true that intercourse is more a physical experience for men and more a sensual and emotional experience for women, it would be logical to assume that sex between two women involves much more talking and touching and much less emphasis on orgasm.

This is true, says Dr. Schwartz.

"Lesbians associate frequent sex with aggression and lack of tenderness as opposed to intimacy, and so they tend to express their intimacy in more passive ways, such as cuddling."

Not all couples fit these gender-based patterns of intimacy and sexuality. Certainly, not all women express their emotions with ease; nor do all men fail to. There are women who can happily indulge in sex without the 'strings' of intimacy, and men who must feel very close to a woman, emotionally and perhaps even spiritually, over an extended period of time, before being ready for physical involvement.

The patterns of sexuality and intimacy I have described are generally true for couples before a life-changing crisis disrupts the balance of their relationships.

At the same time that a woman is grieving after learning she has cancer, her mate also grieves. He, too, is threatened by cancer and loss. Often, because men have difficulty revealing their pain and may have even more difficulty reaching out for help, men face their fears alone.

They certainly don't, and usually can't, talk about these fears with each other and may believe there is no one they can talk to, or who has ever had these problems before.

For all of us, the greatest fear is fear of dying. Right after diagnosis, mates think immediately, "She may be dying.

"I could lose the woman who is my companion, my friend and my lover."

If she dies, so does their collective history and the life they have built together. Losing her means losing part of himself.

And possibly leaving him to raise their heartbroken children alone.

Her body is changed by cancer and the change is a

loss to him, also: of breasts he enjoyed fondling or of her mobility or her ability to have children; of her vitality; of her usual self.

He may fantasize what her body will look like after cancer and cancer treatments change it.

He may fear being repulsed by her new appearance and, worse, not being able to hide that reaction and cause her more pain.

He will be afraid of hurting her emotionally, by saying or doing the wrong thing (or not saying or doing the right thing).

He may be afraid of accidentally hurting her physically, in her post-operative state, particularly during lovemaking. He might think sex will slow healing or cause the cancer to return or that he will develop cancer through sexual contact.

If you cannot express these fears, then you cannot get the reassurance of the truth.

Mates fear causing physical or psychological pain, and they also fear that she will suffer both and they will be unable to help. "My mate's reaction was feeling helpless," many women wrote. In the face of an incurable disease, the pain and discomfort of surgery and treatment as well as the psychological pain of grieving, a feeling of frustration and helplessness is a natural reaction.

If you are a woman with cancer in a relationship, here are the fears your mate will have or could have:

- She may die.
- I might not be able to support her through this.
- I might not be able to accept her changed body.
- She may develop an unhealthy emotional dependency on me, on her doctor, on her caregivers
- She may not be able to do what she used to do (work in or outside the home, contribute to our family income, share activities we used to enjoy)
- I may not be able to meet her needs now; to help her
- I may not be able to suppress my own needs.
- I may lose control (cry, break down)
- I may be powerless to help her
- I may no longer be able to make love to her (I may not have erections when I want them now)
- I may be pushing her to be well before she is ready
- Sex will be impossible/difficult/painful for her now; I must be some kind of monster to want sex now
- She won't want sex; her desire will never return
- How will I help our children understand? How can we be honest with them but also protect them? What if I have to be both mother and

father to them?

- How will we be able to pay for the extra care, medications, treatments, and other costs not covered by our health insurance?
- How can we be sure we are getting the best possible treatment for this type of cancer?
- How will this affect my performance on the job? How can I manage the stress? Will it affect my future in my career? How can I be with her enough, look after our family and still earn our living?
- I am losing my sense of self, my direction, my feeling of security. I have lost her support of my life and career needs.
- She is so ill, so angry, so tired all the time, so irritable. I feel like she is pushing me away; that she doesn't need me.

Your fears will often mirror those of your mate:

- I might die.
- I am mutilated now. I hate my body now – it has failed me. He (she) must be repulsed by me now.
- I need support but my mate may not be able to (want to) give it.
- I may not be able to work again (care for my family, care for myself).
- I am overburdening everyone around me with

my needs; they must resent it.

- We may not be able to have sex again (my desire may never return. Maybe he no longer wants to make love with me).
- When will I be my normal self again?
- Our poor children/relatives/friends – look what I've done to hurt them!
- How will we ever be able to pay for the care and medications?
- How can my mate possibly be coping on the job? How are his co-workers reacting? Do they know? What if he's fired?
- What if I get worse – then will I have to go to a hospital? I want to be at home.
- I am losing control! I may be going crazy! This is more than I can bear!

It's natural for family members, particularly children and husbands, to be protective. At the same time, they fear that they will not be able to help, that their efforts will be insufficient.

In the face of her raw emotional reactions – anguish, weeping, anger and depression, all part of grieving, men fear losing control.

They may see this flood of emotion as a morass which could engulf their family.

Men say they must "be strong" for their partners

while they are grieving. Men feel they must not, ever, "let go." Some even see their duty as constantly urging her to "stay positive" or "cheer up!"

A life-threatening crisis may cause a mate, for the first time perhaps, to contemplate the certainty of his or her own mortality. It also forces him to consider the future.

Men need, during this time, to see themselves as pillars of strength, but to do so, they might need to deny their own pain and postpone their grieving. This can backfire.

Men may feel coerced to be strong soldiers, the backbone of the family during crisis.

Men often try to ignore their own feelings of sadness, to deny their depression, to keep going.

What women see as their mates' denial or emotional withdrawal can, in fact, be a way of masking anxiety and depression.

Several women said that their marriages were "just fine" now, as long as they never mention cancer.

Because their mates would not talk about the cancer or anything connected with it, and insist upon what they call "acting normal," these women could not find out if this was true denial, or if their mates simply did not know what to say and feared saying the wrong thing.

Or perhaps they were embarrassed, particularly if the cancer was gynecologic or of the digestive system. But how could they know, since it was a taboo topic?

In weak marriages where the two have very little communication skills, not talking can very well be denial or even emotional abuse.

Sally's husband would not talk, at all, about her cancer, saying "just go have the operation and get it over with!"

After she did, he said he believed she had invented the cancer. This was the most deeply troubled relationship I encountered.

Most men may, at least for a time, deny the cancer. This temporary denial may be the healthy reaction therapists can emotional distancing, that is temporarily putting off dealing with problems that seem insurmountable.

Mates may inflict pain without ever meaning to.

They sometimes look to someone outside the family for support and understanding, in the belief that their mates already have enough to deal with.

This can happen at the very time that their wives most need to analyze the experience out loud and hear how it is affecting their mates.

Wives may see this stoical behavior from husbands not as sustaining strength but as both denial and rejection.

For any of us, it is excruciatingly painful to see a loved one being hurt. The pain is a private thing. No one else can really enter your pain and your grieving.

For many men, unaccustomed as they are to examining and understanding their emotions, it is an experience they might just as soon skip.

Bobby, the young husband who learned of his wife's cancer during his father's funeral, received a double blow.

He found he could not distance himself.

After initial denial, Sherry wrote, "My husband faced death with me, faced the surgery, handled a quite necessary change of doctors, loved me, got quite angry at me at one point, screamed with me, and at times I hated him more than anyone else in the world.

"Throughout all this, he found out things about himself he didn't want to know, things people don't have to know unless they are pushed to the very edge."

But they, and their marriage, survived.

In his own emotional turmoil, a man naturally looks

to his mate to send him some clues about how to react. How she wants and needs to be treated.

He fears what he sees as pushing her, for recovery or for sex too soon, but he also fears her mood swings, her depressions, her short temper, her rage.

When will she be herself again, he wonders.

He watches for a hint, some signal, some clue that she is not lost in grief, that she is surviving psychologically as well as physically. That she wants to resume sex, that she is still herself.

That they are OK.

Of course, she is not her usual self, not yet and probably not for some time to come. Cancer and recovery – becoming a cancer survivor – does cause some permanent changes emotionally and spiritually as well as physically.

Grief work is not accomplished quickly, and is not completed on any schedule. Survival is individual, not like project management.

Everyone has an increased need for comforting in a crisis, particularly the person at the centre of that crisis.

A person with cancer needs more kindness and affection. She is more vulnerable – perhaps becoming so 'thin-skinned' that she literally has no skin but has become a mass of exposed nerve endings.

When we are seriously ill, we all have an almost childlike need to be cared for. So do the closest people to us (although they will not admit it). In the traditional relationship, where it is mostly the man's contribution to provide material needs and mainly the woman's to minister to the couple's emotional needs, her need to be nurtured now may confuse and disturb her mate.

Therapists call this role reversal. Now, the woman needs her mate to perform her usual nurturing role for both of them, and, if they have children, for them also (and, in addition, for parents, other relatives and close friends).

He is threatened with loss, worried, also grieving, probably physically exhausted because of the changes in their lives and his own need for affection is also increased. Needing to be comforted himself, he may not be able to give his wife the increased affection and support she needs.

Lillian Leiber and her colleagues at E.J. Meyer Memorial Hospital at the State University of New York surveyed the relationships of couples in which either the husband or wife has cancer.

They found that all four groups studied (men and women with cancer, their wives and husbands) had a significantly increased need for affection and the need to show protectiveness toward their mates, an increased desire for physical closeness including simply being together, holding hands, embracing and kissing, and a decreased need for intercourse.

Mary L. S. Vachon, a counselor and research scientist at The Clarke Institute of Psychiatry in Toronto, explained this.

Dr. Vachon says that the desire for more closeness is an expression of love for both a woman and her mate: "The attempt to continue intimacy is life-affirming. I'm not just talking about genital sex, although that is part of it, but the other kinds of intimacy, such as touching, feeling, being with each other. The patient's family and the people who love her must reach out to her, convincing her that they still love her. This is vital!"

Even with this increased need for affection, some women and some spouses do withdraw into their own pain.

Dr. Leiber and her colleagues believe that such withdrawal is relatively rare. They base this conclusion on their study of long-married couples whose ages ranged from 27 to 58.

Dr. Leiber concludes that because the marriages have lasted an average of almost 20 years, the 37 couples studied are probably in happy or at least content and stable relationships.

Withdrawal may be more common in less happy couples with weaker communication skills, say Andrew C. von Eschenbach, M.D. and Leslie R. Schover, both of the Section of Sexual Rehabilitation at M.D. Anderson Hospital in Houston, Texas.[7]

They have written that emotional withdrawal by a woman or her mate is a frequent consequence of the many fears, the depression and the tensions caused by cancer and cancer treatment.

"All this turmoil leaves little energy to devote to sexuality or relationships," they say.

In her confusion and fear, a woman may direct great anger to her partner.

Why do I have to go through all this, she wonders.

How dare he be so calm, so even-tempered, so healthy?

She may displace her own sense of mutilation and self-disgust onto her mate, in effect creating rejection because she expects it.

---

[7] *https://will2love.com/about-us/*

https://en.wikipedia.org/wiki/Andrew_von_Eschenbach

"Bobby sometimes hates me for…" Sherry wrote. There followed a list: crying, being angry or frustrated or too tired. Bobby may be impatient or angered by her reactions, but he has never actually said he "hates" his wife.

That's her assumption.

It is common, Kathleen V. Cairns, a psychologist and teachers who specialized in counseling people with cancer, told me.

Women do project their feelings of inadequacy and self-hatred onto their mates, then punish them for it.

Arlene and John are such a couple who went to Dr. Cairns for help. In their mid 50s, they have been married for almost 30 years.

They have five children, now grown. Both said their marriage was good before cancer. Since her mastectomy, Arlene and John have had what Dr. Cairns calls "severe marital discord."

She noted in her file on this couple:

Arlene feels John is not assisting her recovery, that he rejects her, that he no longer loves her. She says she has approached him sexually and has been rebuffed.

John says she rejected him after her mastectomy and that she is unable to forgive him for his awkwardness and for his ambivalent feelings about her illness and her surgery.

Both wept throughout the first two interviews. Arlene is projecting her own self-hatred and fear onto John, and then she is punishing him for it. She had a female friend in immediately after her surgery so that John would not have to look after her. Now Arlene blames John for her having to make this arrangement. She still refused to allow him to look at her scar, claiming he could not stand seeing it.

Dr. Cairns taught Arlene and John how to tell each other what their needs are.

Over their ten sessions of therapy, Arlene came to see that she had never given her husband a chance to accept her changed body. As it turned out, he was not at all repelled.

Actually, she learned, her husband feels more protective towards her now. As communication was strengthened, their relationship improved and satisfying sex resumed.

In her anguish, a woman can convince herself that it is not possible for her husband to still love her and still desire her. She can make it impossible for him to help her by sending conflicting signals.

If he does want sex, he is being selfish. If not, he no longer desires her, he is heartless. If he does grieve, he is being weak and childish; if not, he is self-centred and uncaring.

Given this situation, a man may begin to feel he can't win.

For both genders, physical and emotional pain reduce or cancel the feelings of arousal. Because of cancer treatment or grieving, a woman may feel weak, or extremely frail, as if her bones are made of spun glass.

She may worry that having sex will harm her or her partner. Desire may have fled, leaving only an oddly numb feeling, even if the cancer did not affect a sexual part of her body.

If it did, sex may be difficult or cause discomfort or pain, or she may now believe intercourse to be impossible, if she has lost her vagina and not has sex therapy to help her find alternative ways of sexual expression.

Many women said that after cancer they could not become aroused for a very long time, or there would be the first stirrings of arousal and then everything would just shut down.

This sudden death of arousal is one of the common signs of depression and of grieving.

It would seem to be the opposite when a woman suddenly has a voracious need for sex, but this is also a frequent reaction to a crisis, especially a brush with death. Sex, like intimacy, is life affirming.

To have sex is to be healthy, normal, totally alive. In bed, she can prove to herself, and her mate, that she survives, that at least one part of her life still works, and that she is still a woman.

Her mate may be equally sexually insatiable, but it is more likely that he will want to avoid sex, because he is unsure of how she is 'really' or he is afraid and depressed himself or he feels guilty for wanting the physical comforting and release of sex.

There are several studies of sex after cancer revealing that, depending on the type of cancer, a woman's prognosis (the likely outcome of cancer, either toward recovery or death) and what sex was like for them before cancer, from 30 per cent to virtually all couples have sexual problems.

Men tend to have difficulty getting or maintaining an erection (called secondary impotence) or may reach orgasm much too soon (premature ejaculation).

Among her clients, Dr. Cairns has found that about half the men suffer secondary impotence after their mates have gynecologic cancer. Dr. Lamont has found in his practice that sex stops temporarily or permanently for one in three couples after the woman has cervical cancer, and for four out of every five couples coping with cancer of the ovaries or vulva.

Because of either their own sexual problems or their concern for their mates, some men tell their wives they don't really care if they do resume sex, saying "Sex doesn't really matter. What I care about is that you are alive."

While these men think they are sending a positive message, as in: "I care about you for far more than your body," in her grief a woman may hear a very different message.

Is he lying, she wonders, or does he no longer desire me and he's trying to spare me the pain of knowing that?

Could he not want sex?

Or could he be having an affair?

He is grieving, and his penis, which is a half voluntary and half involuntary organ, is also grieving. As sex therapists point out, sex is about ten per cent physical and 90 per cent emotional and intellectual. They often say that the brain is the major sex organ.

When he wants to, and cannot, or when she wants him to, and he cannot, sexual problems may add to the couple's tension and distress. This performance pressure, and performance failure, can cause real, long-term impotence. It is reversible, but usually not without help from a qualified marriage counselor or sex therapist.

Performance anxiety is not exclusively a male problem. Women also feel pressure to be 'good' enough.

For women there is the added concern: Am I cheating him of satisfaction? Jennie, an elementary school teacher who had a mastectomy when she was 31, reflected this anxiety when she wrote "At first, it was hard to feel attractive for my husband. I tried to be better at sex. Now, I am just myself."

There is usually a great deal of pressure the first time a couple have sex after her cancer surgery. Both are anxious, both are afraid, both want it to be good. But, like their first time together, when they were dating or on their wedding night, that first time after generally is not a trip to the moon. Here is how women describe it:

"More cuddly, very cautions. Because my surgery was in the abdominal area, we both worried about physical problems. It was very tender as well, because of our new awareness of death and the possibility of losing each other."

– Joy, 31, married her lover of five years two years

after she had cancer

"I was nervous and self-conscious. My husband doesn't appear to see any change."

-- Mabel, 65, in a long-term, happy marriage

They also said it was scary, awkward, funny, touching. If the first time is hard for women married many years (and it is) it is even more difficult for single women who would like to start a new intimate relationship, but fear revealing themselves to a prospective lover.

I remember, with an aching clarity, when I told a man for the first time, a man I cared about and wanted to have a relationship with, about my mastectomy.

One evening, we sat in my apartment, talking.

"There is something I have to tell you about myself," I began tentatively, "and – oh – I am so afraid that after you know, you won't want to see me again. You won't want to know me anymore."

He came to sit beside me, putting a consoling arm around me. "What?" he asked.

So I told him, and, because it was still so soon, I cried.

It was okay, he said, comforting me.

But two days later, he phoned to say "I just can't face

it. I can't face you and what you look like now. I'm sorry."

That summer, he married someone else.

Did I tell him too abruptly?

Explain it all wrong?

Or was he an emotional lightweight who would have collapsed under any difficulty?

Should I could myself lucky?

At the time, I was very hurt, and felt rejected. I decided not to become involved again until I felt more sure of myself and certainly not until I could comfortably tell a man without expecting rejection.

How do you tell a potential lover that you have or had cancer?

"It does impose a great deal of strain on a relationship," Gayle, 25 and single, wrote. "Sometimes, the relationship doesn't survive. How do I tell a new man? Cancer has been such a big part of my life, it usually comes up long before that moment."

"I've only had one relationship since hearing I had cancer," Linda, 33 wrote. "I met him at Sloane-Kettering [cancer centre] in New York, at a group meeting. He said, 'Hi, I'm leukemic,' and I said "Hi,

I'm Hodgkin's.' We laughed, and went from there.

"It was no more awkward than any first time," Jane, 45 and recently divorced, said confidently. "I expect that anyone I would find a serious candidate would be mature enough to accept it."

"I tell a new man as easily as I tell anyone else. It depends on the person, on the expectations. It's not a problem. This is me, I'm not concerned, so why should he be?" This from Barbara, who, at 48, has divorced and gone back to school.

Despite their bravado, it is not easy. But, as one woman pointed out, anyone over 25 has probably earned some honorable scar in his or her life.

Being open about your needs gives him a chance to confide, a good beginning for any intimate relationship.

What about female lovers?

Although I cannot draw conclusions from the few I was able to find or read about, I believe that lovers of women, whether male or female, have the same problems, the same fears of inadequacy and failure, with the exception that a female lover may have a somewhat better understanding of what it means to a woman to lose her breast or her vagina.

"When other people are ill, I care; but with my

lover's illness I suffer. I have felt useless, panic, rage and self-pity. I have and may again pretend, to myself and my lover, strength, boredom, nonchalance... [when what I actually feel is] pain, confusion and fear...I have often not been able to counsel myself out of hiding behind pretense."[8]

While this could easily have been written by a husband, it was actually written by Dinah, who lives with and loves Nancy.

The mere fact that a lover is female does not guarantee empathy, as I learned from another woman.

Meg felt abandoned and pressured by her lover, and although Meg did the leaving, she is hurt and bitter. Here is what she wrote:

"When my lover of eight years found illness frightening and repulsive, she found me frightening and repulsive.... After four months of trying to prove how wonderful I was, despite the pain, I left.

"We didn't know there was another way to think about these things: I was shut in my own silence, trying to behave, to convince her. I was shut in guilt, crazed by it, feeling I had no right to expect anything

---

[8] *Dinah, "Breaking Down the Isolation," Off Our Backs, Off Our Backs, Inc., Washington, D.C., Vol.XI, No.5, May, 1981*

extra from her and needing so much. I was also shut in rage, rage that she could refuse me herself, her solidarity."[9]

Now Meg believes that she and her lover might have stayed together, if only. If only they had talked. Shared their pain and confusion and loss. Realized that other couples have faced this and have worked through it.

That is the subject of the next chapter, but first let's look at what happens when a couple can't work it out.

Although Dr. Pepper Schwartz says that about one in five American women and one in three American men who are beyond age 25 and married have had, or are now having, an affair, none of the women I talked to had, or admitted to, an affair after cancer.

Those who did find new lovers were single or divorced. I expected some women to have affairs, perhaps to prove that they are still desirable or to boost self-confidence, but no one mentioned it.

Dr. Kathleen Cairns confirms that some women have affairs after cancer, but she says it is relatively rare. And many wives fear that their husbands will stray,

---

[9] Meg, "The Solidarity I Needed," *Off Our Backs, Off Our Backs, Inc., Washington, D.C., Vol.XI, No. 5, May, 1981.*

but few do.

In Canada and Britain, one in three marriages ends in divorce. In the States, it is one in two. How can it be that two people exchange their vows of love and commitment, only to part in acrimony and bitterness?

The causes of divorce, experts, say, are complex, but generally they agree that marital breakdown is most likely when:

- there is too little money,
- or a couple can't agree on how to use the money they have;
- when one or both are sexually dissatisfied,
- when they can't talk about their problems and work out compromises
- when they have lost the conviction that they are a team and have reverted to living largely separate lives.

Among the women I interviewed or received questionnaires from, four marriages and two long-term love relationships had ended after cancer.

All but one woman believed that they had separated or divorced because of weaknesses in the relationship that developed long before her diagnosis.

Judging by the remaining woman's story, this was also true in her marriage.

For every one of these women, the cancer and treatment brought increased tension to already troubled relationships, providing not the problem by another problem the couple could not, or chose not to, cope with.

The mostly unspoken agreement between Jennie and Tim was that they would leave the city she loved to live on his family's farm. Jennie would teach grade four in the nearby village, while Tim worked to make the farm profitable.

Although Jennie didn't care for country living, she went along with her husband's plans for several years because this was his dream.

She wanted him to be happy. Eventually, she wearied of teaching and thought of changing careers or perhaps returning to school.

Then, she discovered she had breast cancer and had a mastectomy.

Afterwards, when she shopped for casual clothes that were pretty and feminine and that would also cover her scar and help keep her prosthesis in place, she was disappointed.

The selection in bathing suits was limited; sundresses and lingerie were nonexistent. That discovery led to her new career, designing and making attractive and practical clothing for women who have had a mastectomy.

While Jennie's home business grew, their farm remained a marginal business. A year after her surgery, Jennie and Tim separated. She moved her business to the city, and it has thrived. Relatives blamed the couple's financial problems and her cancer for the break-up of their marriage, but Jennie doesn't see it that way.

"I don't believe I'm the same person now, but my husband doesn't accept that," she wrote. "Now, I put a high value on what I accomplish, but he still can't understand why I didn't stay teaching and why I need to do something to help women who have had a mastectomy."

Jennie's marriage ended not because of her cancer, but because her husband could not accept her revised goals. They'd simply grown into different people, with different goals in life.

Predictably, women who felt deserted by husbands or lovers or who stayed in abusive relationships were the least happy.

Women who divorced and found new goals, including new lovers, were among the most content women I spoke to.

Noreen is one. "Eighteen months after my surgery, my husband again decided he was miserable in our marriage. After a few months of trying to deal with this, we agreed to separate for one year.

"As an alcoholic, he feared for his sobriety of 15 years, and I feared a [cancer] recurrence if I continued in the stressful situation. I have not had a relationship since our separation.

"My mastectomy was not a problem to my husband. He gave me 100 per cent support and loving care. So, cancer was not a factor. My year of separation has been happy and I am unwilling to return to the marriage. Now I am putting myself and my goals first!"

Per also came to a new, more positive view of herself after cancer. Her mate was initially supportive and loving, but that changed.

"I wanted much more from our relationship, and became more demanding, including sexually. But he never touched me sexually again after the operation. Instead, he had an affair – with his right hand. He said he loved me, then he invited me out of the relationship, the bastard!"

"I was devastated that my playmate, the man I supported for 12 years, would desert me. And very angered that after pulling him through so many of his bad experiences, he folded under my crisis!"

Per has moved herself and her business back to her

hometown.

She still sees her ex occasionally. "Now I hire him to change my car's oil. Our relationship is better now, and cheaper.

My life is better, but very lonely. I'm just beginning to accept being alone, reclaiming my self, gaining confidence.

I am going to meet a supportive woman, and we will become lovers."

Single women under 30 tended to expect rejection from some potential lovers, with reason. Men who are immature or who have personal problems such as a history of emotional illness or alcoholism are the most likely rejecters.

Women beyond age 50 also feared being deserted by a long-term mate, seeing their cancer as just another reason for his attention to wander to a much younger woman. But most women in every age group expected their mates to come through for them, and most husbands and lovers deserved this trust.

Those women who were betrayed, particularly if the relationship was long term, were the most likely to be bitter and often had trouble completing their grieving.

Of the women I questioned, 12 per cent lost a mate or

lover. All but three found a new lover/mate. While six said their marriages are even closer than they were before cancer, 20 said their marriages are just as good as they were before cancer.

Clearly, despite the pain, stress and chaos cancer causes, most marriages endure. Most couples cope.

And some grow stronger.

SEVEN

Love Heals

After thirty years of psychoanalytic practice and teaching, I remain convinced that love is still the most powerful human therapeutic agent we have.

- Theodore Isaac Rubin

Recently, I met John, a husband, father and businessman who is president of a small manufacturing company. While making the introduction, our host mentioned that I am a writer and was working on a book.

"Oh," John said with interest, "and what is the book about?" It is about a woman's relationship to herself and to the people in her life, I told him, and what happens in those relationships after she has cancer. John looked surprised for a moment, then shocked.

He quickly changed the subject.

That reaction, of confusion and aversion, was one I encountered often when I told people the subject of this book. I never did learn why John needs to avoid talking about cancer or about people who survive cancer, but I suspect it has to do with the universal fear of illness.

On another evening, at another gathering, I met Francis, a Roman Catholic priest and a born storyteller. He, too, reacted to this book's topic in an often-repeated way, by telling this story recounted to him, he said, by a friend who is a minister: A young couple had worked hard to save for a formal wedding and to furnish their new apartment, and finally it was just a few weeks before their wedding day.

During the last weeks of preparation, the bride-to-be had complained of being very tired, but everyone assumed this was just a matter of wedding planning exhaustion combined with pre-nuptial jitters. To be sure, though, she went to her doctor who did a full check-up, taking blood samples to be sent for testing. The couple were married and went off on a Caribbean honeymoon marred only by the bride's constant fatigue.

The day after they returned home, her doctor got the

lab results showing that she had leukaemia. When he learned the diagnosis, her new husband took his keys and coat and walked out the door. He hasn't been heard from since by his family, friends, boss, minister, or his wife.

This isn't what usually happens, after cancer.

John's reaction of avoidance and Father Francis' story of rejection typifies the most common beliefs about cancer and relationships. Denial and desertion does happen, but all research indicates that it does not happen very often. The most common pattern among couples is that they have trouble in adjusting to the changes cancer brings to their lives and the problems it causes for a period of time, usually from the time of diagnosis until several months to a year or two after treatment is completed.

Most couples emerge from these difficult times feeling individually stronger and more closely bonded to each other.

So here is a real story, of what happened in one relationship after cancer. It is a story not of denial or rejection, but of a couple who did have a hard time but who are, individually and together, survivors.

I am sure there are tens of thousands of couples like Nancy and Don, now even closer after cancer.

Yet in all the years it took to write this book, no one

ever told me anecdotes of couples like them except a few caregivers, most often nurses, and women like Nancy who have lived through cancer and renewal.

Unlike the couple in Father Francis' story, Nancy and Don are typical of couples who are committed to each other, before and after cancer.

Nancy is an attractive, outgoing woman of 50 who has curly brown hair and dresses mainly in neat tailored skirts and colourful blouses.

She is a social worker, but if you have children and watch their television programs, you may have seen Nancy's work. Until a few years ago, she was a professional puppeteer, appearing behind the scenes on many kids' TV shows over the past 25 years.

She and Don, who have three children and one grandchild, recently celebrated their thirtieth wedding anniversary.

In 1985, Nancy found she had breast cancer and elected to have a lumpectomy, followed by radiation treatments.

A year later, a tumour was found in her other breast and she had a second lumpectomy and a second course of radiation treatments. Just a few months later, she told me:

"Before the cancer I had never felt better in my life. I

had a ridiculous amount of energy and was happily studying at university, working as a puppeteer, running my own company and an active household. My biggest battle was not with my physical ability to be active, but with my extreme loss of energy. However, as I still had one very good breast, there was little interruption in my joy of sexual pleasure. There were perhaps three months that my husband and I just tried to recover from the shock of having to face the disease itself. Now he can tell me that at the time he was terrified of losing me and really tried to keep busy so that he didn't have to think about the consequences of the disease too much.

"He did not tell me this at the time. He did try to be extra loving and tender. His support made things much easier for me. I continued with school and I continued to play tennis and swim. I reduced my workload.

"Our lovemaking seemed to be just as frequent and even though I was trying to cope with estrogen withdrawal (she stopped taking hormone replacement also at this time) as well as the radiation effects, I enjoyed the closeness and intimacy because it made me feel safe and secure and gave some semblance of normality to our lives.

"The biggest blow came with the second diagnosis. Neither my husband nor I can remember the four-

INTIMACY

week period following the surgery. Somehow it was so painful psychologically that we have even blotted out the names of some of my doctors and what we did after I got home from hospital.

"Our sex life changed considerably. For a period of time my husband seemed to be impotent most of the time. I had little if any sexual arousal. Often, I would feel the desire, but never had an orgasm during intercourse, and only managed to get relief from sexual tension, when it did infrequently appear, through masturbation.

"Somehow this has become the norm, and it disturbs me a great deal. My own sexual fantasies no longer work for me . . . (because) they merely make me feel sad at the loss of my self-image as a sexy lady.

"My husband tells me that my body does not offend him in any way . . . that he loves me as I am. He has been good about giving me extra affection and has suddenly become a romantic in his old age!

"At one point, he suggested that perhaps my image of myself would improve if I wore a camisole or a lacy shirt when we are making love. I refused the suggestion at the time.

"Then one evening this fall I was too tired to fully undress and put on a nightgown. I just crawled into bed in my underwear, and my husband was very aroused! I am currently trying to make use of this information with only very moderate success.

"I have had several life changes recently (in addition to cancer.) I turned 50, a psychological blow in itself. Then I became a grandmother, which is utterly delightful, but does make one suddenly feel like one has joined an older generation.

"I have started a new job and I continue to work toward my degree. I cannot honestly say that sex is as good for me now, and the thought has crossed my mind that perhaps I should not expect it to be, but I'm not ready to give up yet. Obviously, sex and intimacy are still very important to me.

"Am I happy? In general, yes, very happy. My relationship with my mate is still very good. From some perspectives, the purely sexual aspect, it needs adjustment. But I love him and he loves me. I feel closer to my mate, more intensely aware of each day, focused on my priorities, and eager to live. I feel optimistic about my future!"

Nancy and Don reflect many couples, I found. They did have periods of shock, denial, grief, frustration.

There were small problems to be overcome, and there were problems that were larger and which took much longer to resolve.

Like many couples, Nancy and Don found it difficult

to accept that learning to live with cancer takes time.

Adjustment and acceptance don't come in a matter of days, or even months.

When I looked at the happy couples to see what they did to learn to cope, I found that couples in marriages that survive cancer do these things:

Emphasize what is positive

"What is the key to survival?" I asked on the questionnaire.

Half of those who answered agreed that the essence of survival is in keeping a positive attitude toward life and toward your own worth and the worth of your relationships.

Almost as many women said that love for family and friends are also key to happiness after cancer as well as to survival.

Keeping positive, they said, is focusing on life and living, trusting it, refusing to be bitter.

Remaining hopeful for the future while concentrating on the good things there are in the here and now.

Emphasizing what is strong in your self, your mate, and in your relationship.

I didn't find anyone who feels that she and her mate have mastered this. What matters to them is that they are trying to make the most of every moment and every day.

"When it happened, David and I told each other that we were going to live day by day and get as much enjoyment as we can," Cheryl said, "and it was such a good idea! My God! Let's live for today, have fun! Well, we're doing that, to a certain extent, but this year, with him in school and me supporting us, we've sacrificed a lot. Not too long ago David was saying 'you know, we're not living life the way we should. We should be having more fun!' I agree, we should!" And that lead them to consciously make time for and make plans for family time and couple time.

Talk, about your needs, your fears, your dreams!

Admitting to each other that they should be enjoying their lives more was the first step to finding ways to be happier together for Cheryl and David.

Revealing your feelings and fears reveals who you are as well as what you need to be more fully alive.

In doing so, you're sharing yourself as well as sending a message that says, "I value you enough to let you know me as I really am, weaknesses as well as strengths."

This soul-baring is necessary for intimacy, but it is difficult for many of us, but intimacy is not possible without it. Many couples can get along well with scanty communication skills, until there is a crisis in their lives.

Then, if one person feels a strong need to communicate but the other doesn't (or can't, or feels threatened) the result can be that one uses communication blockers such as the silent treatment or withholding sex, affection, companionship and support.

This leaves the one who wants to talk feeling isolated and rejected.

Not being able to talk to each other is the primary reason for marriage breakdown.

Toni, who is 33, has lived with Mark for seven years.

When they learned she had cancer, she thought of her uncle, who had died of kidney cancer a few years before she met Mark.

"I went to visit my uncle daily. What amazed me was his attitude. I learned so much about the importance of the moment and of acknowledging the people I care about. Life can change so quickly and you cannot afford to put off communicating with the people who are important to you!"

Cathy also wrote about the importance of open communication:

"I suppose I keep getting back to the thing that works best: I keep talking about the things that are important to me; to the people who are important to me."

Form a Partnership to Cope

Cheryl assumed they would continue to deal with their problems as a team, just as they were doing with David's career shift, just as they always had.

But for some couples, forming a team to combat cancer was a more deliberate project. Several women asked their mates to go to doctor or clinic appointments or treatment sessions with them.

Shannon and Peter decided to reject conventional cancer treatment because the hysterectomy doctors recommended would mean that they could never have children.

Instead, they quit their jobs and went looking for an alternative therapy that could save her uterus and cervix and her life.

"I refused hysterectomy and chemotherapy and searched through the alternative healing arts. Together Peter and I travelled through the States and attended several clinics and therapists. I chose fasting, herbal medicines and emotional therapy. In this system, I had to take responsibility for my illness. We tackled my therapy intensively.

"As it turned out, within six months I was in total remission and have stayed in remission for over five years."

"The physicians at the clinic call it spontaneous remission. My friends, my family and I know it was the result of some difficult work."

Shannon is sure her recovery came because of their teamwork in finding and using the treatment they chose.

However, even that success has required adjustment in their relationship, she says, because her mate saw her at her weakest moments, "allowing him an insight that I am not always comfortable with, seeing me being helpless."

Sex also remains a problem for Shannon and Peter:

"It has never returned to the way it was, I think, because of Peter's fear of hurting me."

Despite this, they have grown much closer through their joint project, she wrote, because "My recovery was our goal."

Get the information you need to be well again

Your quest for information starts with your doctor and the people he or she refers you to. Usually, caregivers don't offer information: you must be assertive in asking and may need to push for answers.

You can also learn a great deal by reading (books like this one, online and check libraries and bookstores also).

Some community mental health offices, wellness clinics and community colleges also offer wellness courses, for example, in couple massage, an excellent way to relieve tension and release suppressed emotions.

There are also courses in communication and assertiveness that may help you deal with each other and your caregivers more positively.

While some women I spoke to laud a particular group, others loathed it, which only proves that you need to search out what will work for you.

Nancy Rohleder is one of the women who answered my questionnaire. After her own mastectomy, she felt she wasn't getting the answers she needed from the cancer support groups that existed at the time in her city, so she started AFTER-Mast, a self-help group for women who have breast cancer.

"My own search for answers has been validated by the women who have participated," Nancy wrote. "There are many success stories of women who have overcome enormous difficulties in our group. Obviously, identification is the first bond among us.

AFTER-Mast is a place to talk and share feelings. The opportunity to be a member of a support group should be available to every woman."

Nancy described what happens in one of the meetings, held once a month: "As facilitator, my working agenda includes knowing the questions to ask, reasons for recommendations, talking responsibility for one's own health care, being assertive when necessary, asking for help, sharing strategies for coping, and caring about each other."

In the group, she wrote, women can feel out their options, can exchange information and can overcome isolation.

An added benefit for Nancy is that as a result of AFTER-Mast, she has created a new, challenging and very fulfilling career for herself as a women's counsellor.

I also heard of partner support groups, in which mates had the opportunity to share their concerns with other mates of women with cancer.

One woman who couldn't find a cancer self-help group joined a group for women with major, chronic health problems.

Although she did not get cancer information from other members, she did find the empathy and support she needed, she wrote.

Get help

Margaret was 37 when she realized that something was wrong with her body. Somehow, she says, she knew it was cancer, but she put off seeing her doctor for almost a year because at that time she was steering her family through a different, equally difficult crisis.

Eighteen months earlier, her husband had struck a pedestrian as he drove home. He panicked and fled the scene of the accident.

The pedestrian was seriously injured and Margaret's husband was sentenced to a year in prison, leaving her the sole emotional and financial support of their three children. She left a job she loved for one with a more solid future and a salary that could keep them in comfort and pay her husband's legal bills.

After her husband was released, Margaret finally went to her doctor, who confirmed cancer of the uterus and cervix. She had a hysterectomy.

"I went through a time of deep resentment, of feeling like half a woman. My husband and I talked about it. Although he was very supportive, the issue was how I felt about myself. He could not separate my feelings about me from his feelings about me and his support of me. We couldn't resolve it, so we went to family counselling, which helped us a great deal. Most of all, it helped me to see me."

Couples counselling is not like psychoanalysis: it is less time consuming, does not look to the past to describe current problems, and there are usually positive results almost immediately.

Nancy and Don, the couple at the opening of this chapter, went to marriage counselling because they could not solve their sexual difficulties.

Their counsellor helped them examine their fears and their false expectations, Nancy wrote: "It was the most frightening period of my life. Without professional help, I would not be as mentally healthy as I am now! Our sex life has improved tremendously!"

Competent, caring therapy may be offered through your cancer centre, or you may have to seek a referral from your oncologist or gynaecologist.

Or look in the phone book or online under:

- The Gynaecology/Obstetrics or Oncology Department of a teaching hospital
- State or Provincial psychological licensing association
- Local, state or provincial mental health association
- State or provincial association of medical social workers

- Planned Parenthood or your local women's wellness clinic

Ask for a referral to a therapist experienced in counselling people with cancer or people who are physically-challenged.

Or phone a cancer information hotline.

Most marriage therapists are psychiatrists or gynaecologists and therefore also doctors or psychologists or they are social workers or nurses with advanced training in counselling. Your therapist should also be willing to consult with your doctors.

Questions you should ask a prospective therapist, and answers he or she should give:

Q. How much experience do you have?
A. At least three years.

Q. What approach will you use in our treatment?
A. You talk and I listen. We consider your problems together and look for new approaches to the problem. I can also teach you coping skills.

Q. How long will treatment take?
A. One or possibly two sessions a week for eight to twelve weeks.

Q. Is there homework?
A. Yes. There are exercises in communication and in

sexual relating you and your mate will do at home between sessions.

Q. What are the goals of this therapy?
A. We will make specific goals for our time together during our first session.

Q. Does my mate have to participate?
A. It is best if you work together for positive change in your relationship. However, if your mate refuses to attend, I can help you with self-image and self-confidence issues.

You may be able to join a therapy group or see a counsellor while still at your cancer centre.

If so, these services are part of the cost of your care there. Otherwise, your medical insurance may cover all or part of the cost.

Some counsellors also offer sliding scale rates.

Your best choice is a person you can trust and feel you can work with. It helps very much if they are familiar with your type of cancer and treatment and have an understanding of the particular physical and emotional problems cancer causes us and our mates.

If you do not feel you can trust your counsellor after an initial meeting, ask to be referred to someone else.

What must you contribute to your therapy?

Mainly, you talk, and your therapist listens and makes specific suggestions for change.

You do not have to tell everything about yourself, although withholding information relevant to your problems may slow down treatment or make it impossible. You are expected to sincerely commit yourself to working with your partner and therapist to identify the problems in your relationship, to accept that the only workable solutions lie in compromise and to attend all the sessions and follow your counsellor's recommendations, including doing the homework.

What can you expect to gain from counselling?

Counsellors teach couples how to relate to each other honestly, how to hear what the other is saying, how to negotiate for positive change.

They do not supply ready-made answers. Rather, they teach ways of finding your own answers, of discovering what you both want now and of charting ways to get the things you want and need.

They do this by providing:

1. Information

How your body works and what to realistically expect from it now, after cancer; better ways to communicate; replacing myths about cancer and relationships with truth, having realistic expectations of yourselves and your relationship.

2. Permission

To let go of grief and anger and other hurts from your past; to let go of myths that may be impeding your recovery including sexual myths such as performance anxiety such as the myth that you have to 'give' each other an orgasm every time you make love and to show emotions including love, how to relax and how to accept.

3. Rational views

Helping you counter irrational beliefs and fears, such as "How could he possibly love me now? He couldn't, therefore he must not" which are based on low self-esteem.

Usually, because cancer also threatens a woman's sexual self-image and often causes sexual problems for her and her mate, couples counselling also includes sex therapy.

In sex therapy as in marriage therapy, you learn new ways to relate to each other.

There are no sex surrogates, and you will not be asked to undress, unless the counsellor is a physician doing a routine examination, nor will you be observed having sex with your mate. Progress is judged by the goals you meet, just as in any form of therapy.

Dr. Kathleen V. Cairns, a sex therapist and educator, told me, "Almost everybody worries about intercourse and forgets that their entire body is sexual."

Sexual and sensual pleasuring do not depend on a vagina and a penis, she said, but on two people who care enough about each other to find ways to be loving. Author Michele Landsberg put it even more simply when she wrote, "Sex involves the whole body and the whole heart."

Redefine your goals!

When Shannon and Peter asked themselves what was most important to them, they decided it was: one, Shannon's recovery from cervical cancer and two, having a child.

They focused all their energy on these two goals. During her treatment, Shannon became pregnant.

"I thought that if I could not get my cancer into remission, I would never have a child of my own.

"As a young teenager, I had become pregnant and had allowed my family and others to pressure me to have an abortion although my own ethics were against it. My anger towards myself over this festered for years. I decided that I wanted a child and proceeded to try to get myself healthy enough just to get pregnant and to do the therapy afterwards. I found a physician who thought that it was feasible and he assisted me.

"As it turned out, within six months I was in total remission and pregnant!" Shannon and Peter now have two healthy children, and Shannon has passed the five-year survival anniversary without a recurrence.

Every woman and her mate are concerned during pregnancy; wondering if the baby is healthy, it if has the right number of fingers and toes, if you both are doing all you can do to help your child get a healthy start in life.

After cancer, there are additional worries.

Could your chemotherapy or radiation treatments in the past harm your child now? Probably not, experts say. If you are currently pregnant, cancer treatments could harm your unborn child, depending on the type of treatment.

This could lead to you and your mate being faced with the agonizing decision of whether to abort your child and proceed with treatment, trading that life for the chance to save your own; or to postpone your treatment until after birth and risking your life for that of your unborn child's.

It was once believed that the hormones created by a woman's body in abundance during pregnancy possibly spur any undiscovered tumour to spread and thus reduce her chance of survival, but experts no longer believe this to be true.

And it is now possible to test tumours for their sensitivity to hormones, but this test, called a hormone assay, is one you must request at the time of your biopsy or cancer surgery.

Chemotherapy and radiation treatment to the pelvic area can destroy your ability to become pregnant after treatment has ended.

If you hope to have a child and must undergo pelvic radiation, ask to have your ovaries surgically moved behind your uterus and out of the target area.

After treatment, if you can conceive, the chemotherapy or radiation you had is not likely to affect the health of your baby.

A pregnancy after treatment for cancer is not considered elevated risk, although doctors recommend that you wait to become pregnant until at least a year after your chemotherapy or radiation treatments are completed.

There are only a few studies of pregnancy and

cancer. I encountered some doctors who could not believe that any woman and her mate would even consider a pregnancy after cancer.

How much of a risk is pregnancy, after cancer? It isn't a risk, and this is not a recent finding.

From 1930 until 1965, M. Vera Peters, M.D., a radiation oncologist at Princess Margaret Hospital in Toronto, studied women who had breast cancer and were or subsequently became pregnant.

She concluded that a woman's chance of survival is not affected by pregnancy.

For women who were diagnosed just before or during pregnancy, Dr. Peters, working with James William Meakin, M.D. found that women do just as well, or better, if their treatment is delayed until after the baby is born.

Another encouraging discovery: the five-year survival rate was the same among women who became pregnant after breast cancer and women who did not, but the women who had a child after cancer were much less likely to have a recurrence of their cancer.

This led Dr. Peters and Dr. Meakin to conclude, "pregnancy does not appear to have any detrimental effect on the malignant process and usually adds to the happiness and security of the patient."

Pregnancy may, they said, actually contribute to a woman's survival!

But is it safe for you to have a baby after having cancer?

There are still some doctors who advise against pregnancy for cancer survivors, but their number seems to be dwindling.

All six doctors I asked this question of agreed that pregnancy following cancer should be encouraged.

Walter Rider, M.D., Head of Radiation Oncology at Princess Margaret Hospital, told me, "In the more than 30 years that I've been treating women for cancer, I have never seen a case where the pregnancy was complicated by the fact that a woman had breast cancer before she was pregnant."

If you cannot conceive or bear a child, or chose not to risk pregnancy, but feel your life is incomplete without children, you still have options.

One, adoption, probably would have been closed to women who had a potentially fatal disease in the recent past, but adoption policies have been liberalized.

To find out if a woman who had cancer could adopt, I posed as a potential adoptive parent.

I learned that legal adoption agencies set their own

policies and that all legitimate agencies, public and private, assess prospective parents as individuals with the primary concern being for the well-being of the child.

Your local Children's Aid, Catholic Children's Aid, Jewish Family and Children's Services and government child welfare officials and your doctor, minister, priest or rabbi and lawyer can provide more information on legal adoption policies in your province or state and may also refer you to an adoptive parent support group.

Children don't necessarily bring couples closer or save a failing relationship. If anything, children put more strain on both partners.

But for couples like Shannon and Peter, they also enrich life immeasurably. Inviting children into their lives was not the only couple goal that worked to bring the couples I found closer together.

Cheryl and David decided to spend Saturday afternoons with their daughter, going antique-hunting, on picnics, anywhere away from the phone and his studies. Another couple bought a home and their goal was to renovate it, doing all the designing and most of the labour themselves.

Focus on each other

Couples whose relationships are strong did simple

loving things together and for each other, often renewing the bonds they had forged early in their relationship.

Many women told me that they and their mates had forgotten about the things that gave them pleasure when they were first dating, but that since having cancer these couples have consciously remembered what first attracted them to their mates.

Now they concentrate on these good qualities. They recalled what they had enjoyed doing when they first met, and then considered why they had stopped doing those things.

Perhaps the reason was not enough time, the children, and the cost. Then they rearranged their priorities, sometimes actually scheduling in these shared activities on their calendars.

They made time for fun.

One family I heard of made it a new rule that they'd turn off their phones, order in pizza and play pool every Thursday evening. It was their quality time together.

Fun could be a weekend away, or a picnic with the kids. The activity, women said, didn't really matter as much as that there was only one goal, enjoyment. Worries were left behind.

Play is healthy but most adults have forgotten how to do it, say psychologists James Halpern and Mark A. Sherman.

"Everything we adults do seems to need some rationale, some functional justification. If we stand on a corner, it is to wait for a bus. If we lie on the beach, it is to get a suntan. Why do we have to justify everything we do? Play is something to be engaged in for its own sake -- just for the fun of it."

Sometimes, this fun is sexual.

Remember what sex was like in your first year together?

Why did it change?

Now think further back, to being a teenager and to the fun you had with your boyfriend in the back seat of his car, or later, at your lover's apartment, or perhaps while you were on a camping trip together, lying under the stars.

What made those times hot? How can you recapture that now, with your mate?

Joy, who is 24, married her lover two years after they discovered she had cancer.

Just after their wedding she wrote, "I think we had the feeling that if we, and our relationship, could survive this, we could survive anything. Our relationship is happy and strong. Sex is more adventurous. Having fun has grown to be important to us."

Take the emphasis off sex role stereotypes and value each other as people and as individuals!

Women aren't necessarily the gender more suited to intimacy any more than men are born with a gene for car maintenance, but believing this myth can limit our relationships and our happiness with each other.

Joseph LoPiccolo, Ph.D., a psychology teacher at Texas A&M University and author of **Becoming Orgasmic: A Sexual Growth Program for Women**, says that it is the very traditional couples, those who believe in separating women's work from men's work, for example, who are most likely to have relationship problems.

If we can stop concentrating on what women do, or are "supposed" to do, need or want, and what men do (need/want) and concentrate on what people need, "we would all have a lot better emotional and sexual lives" Dr. LoPiccolo says.

We can enjoy the differences between men and women without using them as an excuse to limit each other.

Who does the dishes or figures out the tax return or changes the baby or does the sexual inviting is far less important than the fact that one of you does, according to Dr. LoPiccolo.

Men and women are much more alike than we are different, once the societal myths are shed. We are precisely alike in our basic needs; for air, water, food, shelter and clothing, love, achievement and sexual release.

Men are no different than women in their emotional needs; for attention, affection, understanding, acceptance and intimacy.

And the sexes are much more alike than different in the fulfilment of these needs, as Masters and Johnson and several other researchers and caregivers point out. It is only social expectation and ignorance, the province of myths, that polarize us.

Remember Nancy and Don?

They are the couple whose sex life almost withered away after her second mastectomy. A year after she filled out the questionnaire, I wrote to her, asking how life is for them now.

Her response was enthusiastic, full of current satisfactions and future plans. This is what she wrote about her marriage: "We did go to counselling, and it helped us. Both my husband and I have become aware, just in the last few months, that we have been slowly recovering from depression. This was a depression so subtle that I don't think we were aware that we were still depressed.

"But now, what a difference there is in our approach to life! This is just in the last few months! We can see we are on this side of the wall! Our sex life has improved tremendously, our energy levels have improved, our plans for our future have suddenly taken shape, and we feel more strongly bonded than ever before.

"I could not believe that his depression over my cancer affected him so strongly, but I suppose I was too busy with my own depression to be able to see his."

It took the help of a therapist, time, and partners making the effort to empathize to help them build a stronger, happier and more sexually fulfilling relationship, Nancy said.

It was not until several months after her radiation treatments ended that both partners could discover the healing in themselves and in their relationship.

We do not have the right to choose what tragedies will change our lives. We can only choose how we will react to these life accidents and what we will learn from them. These crises are not the exception to life, but a part of the tapestry of our lives.

We cannot avoid loss and pain. We can overcome

these setbacks by learning, or re-learning, to trust and to love ourselves and the people we choose to share our lives.

Intimacy is not a cure for cancer, nor for the sorrow it causes, but it can do a lot to mend the damage done. It provides an oasis of peace in our lives, giving us the strength we need to be totally alive.

Though there are many substitutes for intimacy: drugs, alcohol, overeating and overwork are a few; none of these have the healing power of love that is shared.

Love is what makes survival, both terrible and wonderful, worthwhile.

EIGHT

Other Intimacies - Family, Friends and Children

Families, like marriages, have their own complexities and agendas in place long before cancer arrives. Each family, like each woman, must find its own path through trauma.

Just as there is no job description for the grief work each of us must do, there is no one correct way for families to share the burden of their fear and anguish.

When Toni discovered she had cancer, she did not want her parents at her bedside, even though they are a close family:

"My hospital room was inundated with flowers, cards, balloons, not to mention loads of phone calls and visitors. I was absolutely overwhelmed with the good wishes, love and caring that came my way."

It was not until after she went home from hospital that, at Toni's insistence, her parents flew to the West Coast from their home in Boston.

"Their reaction was one of deep sadness, fear and most of all, helplessness. I believe because of the physical distance between us, their shock and anger and devastation were even more magnified. Later, I learned they could not eat or sleep or even share their heartache verbally to each other at that time. There were constant phone calls to me while I was in hospital." The day she was discharged they arrived at her apartment.

"My mother was very hurt at my asking them to come after, but I insisted. I felt it was the best for me.

"My father agreed with my wishes, though I know he wanted to just drop everything and come. Basically, my family and friends had the need to see me, just to make certain that I was the same person I was before the surgery.

"Now, people treat me differently than before. They seem to see me as someone special. They give me gifts and cards when they wouldn't normally do so."

Toni grew up in a happy home, the much-loved youngest daughter.

"My parents raised me without expectation, with unconditional love. They have always accepted me as I am. It wasn't until now that I've been conscious of that."

So why did she initially push away such loving parents at a time when she most needed their support? Looking back, it seems to Toni that she was trying to protect them.

"My biggest problem has been the impact that cancer has on my family and on Mark, my lover. I cannot imagine what my reaction would be if one of my sisters or my brother had it instead of me. It's so much easier being the patient, I think, than the loved one of the patient. As the patient, I know how I feel and I know as much about my health care as I can. I know cancer is something I can beat. Trying to understand the feelings of those I care most about has been a big hurdle, and I am still learning."

While they cannot share your physical pain, the people around you suffer emotional pain very much like your own.

Usually, they try to hide this pain from you. They are also worried, angry, doubting of their ability to help you while feeling that life is suddenly spinning out of control.

They may blame themselves for "allowing" cancer to

happen while, at the same time, blaming you for somehow bringing this misery upon yourself and rearranging everyone's life.

In some families, some family members may find that living with someone with cancer is so agonizing, they'd rather be grieving your death. When they realize this, they can suffer agonies of guilt.

To cope, they also need information and emotional support, which often is inadequate or unavailable. Cancer always has more questions than answers. This uncertainty causes more pain for everyone around you.

So they look to you, the woman in the bed who is grieving and recovering from surgery or ill from chemotherapy or radiation treatments, to help them understand and help them accept.

While they look for this emotional mothering from you, they may also be trying to nurture you, as best they can.

While they may believe they are caring for you, you may feel they are treating you like a helpless child, thus creating additional tensions. Even in close, loving families, during such an emotion-charged time there can be resentments and misunderstandings.

Kathy Smith, R.N., a nurse-clinician at Henderson

General Hospital's Gynaecologic Cancer Clinic in Hamilton, Ontario, explains.

"Patients say all the time that they can accept what is happening to them. But it is their families they feel they have to take care of. Usually, they don't have the energy to take care of everyone else and themselves.

"Also, usually they can't really talk about their own feelings to their mates or their families. They need other people; nurses, counsellors, their friends. I and the other nurse-clinicians do exams and patient education, but most of what we do for patients is listen to what they are feeling, tell them these feelings are normal and act as a family liaison."[10]

They explain cancer and treatment, listen, and are also "positive for today" for people with cancer and their families.

For friends and family without support from caregivers the pain can become unbearable. One escape is to retreat into denial.

After learning she had cancer, Linda, who is divorced, could no longer work and had no option but to move back home, at age 32. Sadly, neither of her parents could help her face her cancer and the

---

[10] *http://www.jcc.hhsc.ca/body.cfm?id=73&fr=true*

losses it caused. Both fled, her mother physically, her father psychologically.

"I told my mother first. I thought that she would be more receptive. Also, since I had lost my only child, I could understand what she might be feeling and I thought I could comfort her. And I needed her to comfort me.

"At first, she seemed to be very understanding. But a month later she just freaked. She visited me at Sloane-Kettering (cancer centre) and said she'd be back at Christmas. Then she went to the Orient, and sent me a cable saying she couldn't deal with it. Said she was sorry. Said she knew that I was strong and I would be fine.

"My father is an alcoholic, and he has denied the situation for eighteen months now, even though we live in the same house! My younger sister is really the only family member that I occasionally talk to about cancer, but she lives 3,000 miles (4,828 km) away. As far as I know, my ex-husband doesn't know."

It would seem that Linda is very much alone.

A woman who has suffered so many tragedies and disappointments could understandably be depressed, or even bitter, but Linda's letter was full of hope and compassion.

The reason, she says, is because of the loving support

of her friends. But friends, like parents and family, don't always come through.

Almost every woman told of losing a friend, but added that they had gained other, better friends after cancer.

Linda: "Some friends changed their opinion of me, but most changed the way they reacted to me, to Linda. The ones that disappeared were usually the ones that insisted on knowing everything at once and the ones who professed to understand right from the first hearing. You think maybe they really do understand. Then you don't see them again."

Friendship is very much like marriage.

Both types of intimacy require kindness and humour, compassion, trust and mutual respect. In both we reveal our most private selves and our needs, feelings and desires.

Not all friendships operate on such an intense level.

There are friends you play tennis with, friends you only see at the gym or when you visit the folks back home or you haven't heard from in years, but you wish well. And there are the friends who know you and like you, just as you are. You could tell them anything.

Just as no one person can fill all our needs, no one

friend can be everything we need her or him to be.

Inevitably, some friends and family members disappoint.

Some have never developed coping skills, have never faced any sort of crisis and have scant resiliency or have never confronted their own vulnerability to such a crisis and to death.

So, like Linda's parents, they flee.

This is not betrayal, but it can feel like it is.

Sherry: "My friends were confused; frightened. For some the fear took over. They stayed away. Others were angry at me. They needed me. 'Be tough!' they said. 'Be strong!' 'Be better.'

"One close friend went through the motions but refused to let me touch her.

"Those friends who continued to treat me as before, with total support, those who did not pretend life was at a standstill because I had cancer, they were most helpful. I closed up pretty tight but I always knew they were there. At the time, I felt I was losing people left and right. But now I see I did not. The friends I lost, in retrospect, were not people I was surprised to lose. My good friends are my better friends now.

"And my mother was magnificent! We have had

quite a stormy life together, but she concentrated on caring for my young son. She was great!"

Often the last people to learn of our cancer are our children.

Some people believe it is too serious and painful a topic to share with children, so they say nothing or they cover up the truth and the seriousness of having cancer.

Children are rarely fooled. Even babies feel the tension and see the worried faces.

Children notice disrupted schedules, sudden silences, people crying or trying not to and they overhear conversations. Because they are so totally reliant upon their families, they are very good at reading the signals and interpreting emotions.

They can read the non-verbal messages of pain and distress. Being excluded does not cushion reality for people at any age.

Instead, it makes them fear the worst, especially if they know they're being lied to.

Young children fear:

- Losing you. That you may go to the clinic one day and never come back.
- Being abandoned by you and by other adults.

- That they may have caused your cancer, because they didn't clean their room or do their homework or get an A on a test.
- That something is very wrong and you are pretending it isn't and treating them like a baby who can't understand.
- That other children will tease, bully or reject them because of your cancer.
- That their real mother is gone and you are a stranger who acts like their mother but doesn't look like her or smell like her.
- Sadness and pain, particularly in families where these emotions are hidden from children.

In addition, older children and teenagers fear:

- That you will desert them, either emotionally, because you are sick all the time, or that you will die.
- That their developing need for independence conflicts with the family's need to draw closer now and face the crisis together.
- That they may lose emotional control, especially at school or in front of their friends.
- That you are withholding information, particularly if it is bad news.
- That they will get cancer, because you have it.

Like you, they may also feel:

Angry

They, like you, ask why this disruptive illness had to happen to their family, and resent having to change or cancel their plans, for example, to accommodate treatment appointments.

Guilt

For their sadness and anger, and for wanting to continue activities with their friends. For just wanting their lives back, as kids or teens. For resenting your needs.

Cheated

Of activities they can't enjoy now because cancer intervenes, for example, cancelled vacation plans.

Helpless

Unable to help you or to assume new responsibilities at home.

Cancer is hard for families, and especially hard in dysfunctional families or families already struggling with other issues, such as poverty.

Marti is divorced.

Until her diagnosis, she was a working single mother. While in hospital her son, then 10 years old, and daughter, eight, stayed with their father, who told the children that their mother had the flu!

Marti described an evening with her children not long after her diagnosis:

"It was early evening, just after dinner. I decided to take a bath and my daughter, Lauren, wanted to come in with me. So we poured in some bubble bath to make it more fun. As the bath went on I sensed that my son was hovering outside the door. We were singing in the bath and the bathroom was completely steamed up.

"We heard the door open slowly and Sean entered, very silently. He started to sing too. We said 'Hi, Sean!' from behind the curtain. Then there was silence.

" I pulled the curtain to get out a while later, and through the mist we saw a note written in steam on the mirror. It said 'I love you Mummy. Sean.'

"I began to cry. Slowly, the door opened again and he peeked in. The three of us stood there and hugged.

"Later that evening, we were all in my bed. While we were lying there, Sean asked me what was wrong. So I asked him and his sister if they knew what cancer is. They said 'Tommy's mother died of that.' My response was 'Well, I'm not going to die.'

"Then I told them about what cancer is, about the bad cells and the good cells. I said that with help I was going to make the bad cells go away."

You may wish there were some magic words to banish your child's fears and confusion and help him or her smile again.

You may wonder if you are telling enough -- or too much. But the actual words you use don't really matter all that much.

What is important is that you want to include your child in what is happening; that you want to help him or her understand and cope, that you are willing to listen to his concerns and answer questions.

Children are remarkably resilient, given the opportunity. Even very young children can adjust to almost anything except rejection.

By sharing your tears as well as your information, you show your child that it is okay to grieve, and it's good to offer each other comfort.

In doing this, you also demonstrate your love for them and respect for their feelings.

When you tell your children about your cancer and how you feel about the changes it is making in your lives, the actual words you choose are less important than the way you say them. Together, sharing a hug and a quiet moment, as Toni did, is best.

It is okay to admit that there are things you don't know.

Saying, "I'm sure we'll all be just fine" is not honest. You can't know this; no one can know exactly how your cancer journey will unfold. It also denies feelings of anger and sadness.

On the other hand, saying, "No one knows for sure" or "You know, there are times I wonder about that, too" is more truthful and it helps lessen anxiety.

Rae Ellen Stager is a registered nurse who had breast cancer. Her son, Ross, was six and very curious when she had her mastectomy. Ross wanted to see the scar but Rae Ellen hesitated about allowing this, concerned that the sight of her scar could cause Ross additional fear and confusion.

She and her husband, a psychologist, finally decided that their son's fantasies about what had happened to his mother's body were probably much more frightening than the reality.

They waited until the incision had healed and carefully prepared their son for what he would see.

His reaction surprised them.

"Gee Mum," he said, "you look just like me on that side." But later that day, and many times over the following weeks, Ross went to his mother and, while gently stroking her cheek, said, "I bet you really feel bad that you only have one breast. I bet you wish that you could have the other one back again. Don't you feel bad about that Mummy?"[11]

You may find your child's questions hard to take, especially while coping with treatment and all the other upheaval.

It may help to tell your mate, close relatives and perhaps your child's teacher what answers you are giving. Part of a child's repeated questioning is for information, and to answer questions children may not be able to ask, such as "Did you get cancer because I behaved badly? Is it somehow my fault?" and "Will I get cancer too?"

The repeated questioning is also for reassurance that you are still you; not, as some children fear, someone masquerading as their mother, that you love them and continue to care for them and that things are normal in their world.

Many women said they drew great strength and felt an outpouring of love from their children, particularly from very young children, which helped sustain

[11] *Gordon L. Stager and Rae Ellen S. Stager, "Sexuality and Cancer," in Margot Tallmer, et al., Sexuality and Life-Threatening Illness, Charles C. Thomas, Springfield, Illinois, 1984, p. 78.*

them during their darkest moments.

Even when there was a kind and supportive mate (and every mate had his or her moments of being unable to provide kindness and support) women turned to their children for a different, simpler intimacy.

Marti: "Now, while I recover, I am home with my children. They have given me strength. Needing to be here for them gives me self-healing energy! And lots of hugs that keep loneliness away!"

Donna: "My older son was ten when I told him I had cancer. He said in shock 'But that's incurable!' So, I explained all I knew and hoped about cancer and how it is not at all incurable. I tried so hard to allay his fears about my death that I put to rest many of my own fears at the same time.

"My younger son was three. He still to this day, though he has seen me naked with scars raging where my breasts once were, he still thinks of me having two breasts like other women."

Sherry: "Lying in that hospital, it was my son's face, his needs, his pain that I healed for. As soon as the anaesthesia wore off, they let him see me. He is just seven, but he acted big and strong for me. He has saved (demanded) my sanity and he has sustained me.

"He has forced me to be more than I am, stronger than I am, and I have seen flashes of the man he will become."

One interesting finding revealed on the questionnaires was that women reported that their daughters "understood" about their cancer, but they didn't elaborate.

However, they described their efforts to help their sons accept cancer in detail, as if they assumed a female child could easily understand and accept, but a male child couldn't without significant effort from them.

While Ann was in hospital for her first chemotherapy treatment, "My husband told our girls I had Hodgkin's disease, and he also told them it is a form of cancer, because we didn't want them to hear it from other children at school.

"What my daughters really wanted to know was 'How did you get it?' So, we explained the disease and the treatment.

"I think it was more traumatic for them that I was in hospital, because neighbours and friends were very kind. They took them for dinners and weekends, and the girls enjoyed it, but it was tiring for them.

"Since I've been home, things have been quieter, but

my husband says that I seem to be more strict with the children. Like their rooms. Always messy. That wouldn't have bothered me so much before.

"A classic line from our younger daughter: she had hurt her foot slightly while we were on vacation, and I wanted her to hurry, someplace we were, and so I said 'Come along, Miss Hop-a-long!'

"She was quite indignant. She said, 'Mum, that's not very nice! I don't call you Mrs. Cancer!'

"I know when I tell her she said that, when she's an adult, she'll be appalled, but I just laughed."

Is there a danger in sharing too much with your child, particularly if that child is very young?

Psychologists say disclosure may hurt your child if you expect her to react as an adult would, have the insights of an adult, or offer you the support that you would expect from another adult.

Very young children understand your need for physical comforting, as in "Mummy hurts" without really comprehending cancer's threats.

It's good for you to turn to your children for affection, just as you offer them extra affection and attention now, but is overburdening a child to expect him to be your confidant, according to Dr. Stan Kutcher, a psychiatrist at Sunnybrook Medical

Centre in Toronto.

You may tell your child you are tired and need quiet time together, or you need a hug, but to tell him how angry you are with your doctor, or wonder aloud what your next blood test or scan will show is to burden him or her with problems beyond a child's level of understanding and tolerance.

Children and teenagers react as we all do. They, like you, may be resentful, afraid, angry, or perhaps revert to some childish behaviour.

Others may become pensive or withdrawn. We each grieve in our own ways, at our own pace.

Even adult children can react in ways that may seem infantile, even bizarre. When Sally, who is 49, told her adult daughter the results of her biopsy, "She turned her back and left the room. It took her three days before she would talk about it, to urge me, very coldly, very unemotionally, to have surgery.

"Later, she said she could get something for me, 'But what's the use, you're dying,' she said. And she laughed!"

What makes this daughter's reaction particularly grotesque is that Sally is a nurse and her daughter is a doctor.

Fortunately, her son, then 23, was better at coping

and therefore better able to help Sally. "He was very supportive, open, honest with his feelings and he listened to my gut feelings," she said.

Elena, a college professor, had long since divorced when she had her mastectomy. She believes she owes her emotional survival to her youngest child.

"The doctors told my children; I was in a state of shock. The middle one couldn't talk about it, and he still finds it difficult, but he just sat and held my hand.

"My older son was supportive but he didn't want to listen; he would just say 'I know you're going to be all right, Ma,' but my daughter was wonderful. She was only 16 at the time. I don't know if I could have gone through it without her. She seemed to be the only person I had that really understood, that I could count on to understand, and that would tell me what I needed to hear at the time that I needed to hear it.

"For example, I was really depressed and there were days when all I could do was lay on the sofa. I really didn't want to be that way, but I couldn't help it. I needed someone to say 'Hey, look, you've got to cut it out now, you've got to quit. Come on, let's get up and go shopping or go out to dinner!' and my daughter would do that at the time when I needed it. If I needed to talk something out, she would listen.

She was there for me!"

Although every woman told of a least one family member or friend who reacted negatively, every woman said she gained friends.

After initial problems, most children came to some degree of understanding and acceptance and could help their mothers both emotionally and by taking on more responsibility on the home front.

Generally, family patterns after cancer tended to be the same as before, but some women found cancer pushed them to work to improve family relationships.

Sharon is one. She decided that she could no longer accept her family's "closed door" policy and finally confronted them. Her risk paid off.

Sharon grew up in a family that was emotionally closed, and for her "the biggest hurdle was getting my family, particularly my mother, to accept me as a whole person again. We don't live near my parents, so I couldn't ask them to go to counselling with me, but when we were together I told them I couldn't keep the doors of my feelings closed any longer. And so my parents finally talked about their fears."

A few women did insist that their parents share their feelings.

Marti wrote, "One thing I had never done was to ask my father for a hug or to tell me he loves me. So, when I finally did, he explained that his love for me is very strong and deep. He just doesn't show it."

This revelation brought Marti to the realization that she must "accept people as they are and not for what I want them to be. Not to expect them to supply what I thought they should give me, rather than what they have to give."

Now, she can accept her father as he is, assured of his quiet, undemonstrative love.

Crisis can be a force leading to the strengthening of families, forcing them to learn to talk to each other, trust each other, come together.

Many women were surprised when formerly untested reserves of strength and love were revealed, as Sally was with her son and Marti with her father. The methods that help couples cope also help families get through tough times.

"My husband and I did a lot of reassuring to friends, family and our children," Noreen wrote. "That attitude created a positive atmosphere. I don't think I lost any friends. I educated them, accepted their offers of help, made them feel better for helping, and became much closer to them and to my son and daughter who took me to chemo and sat with me. It was a meaningful time for me and for them."

Sherry kept what she calls a "killer pace" before cancer, with two jobs, night school to finish a degree, writing and volunteer work, the price for a more challenging and exciting future career.

But after she answered my questionnaire she wrote to say that she had decided to put her career on hold.

"I've cleared two months of summer to be with my son and teach him algebra," she said. It's unlikely that her son, who is seven, really needs training in algebra.

Like many women, Sherry is making an opportunity to be with her child and her mate, to become what Sharon called "more family-centred." Or, put another way, she has reduced life to the essentials to give herself the time, space and family love she needs to heal.

"What is sure is now," Sherry wrote. "I have a son who I must build up, make strong, give my best to. I have treated him like a friend ever since he was conceived. And he is my friend now. Today, there is a quiet over me that I have never known before. I am more real than I have ever been."

NINE

Advanced Cancer - Time enough to say good-bye

One day, while waiting to see your doctor, you may overhear nurses discussing the contents of your chart.

Or it may seem to you that the people at your cancer centre have begun to treat you differently. Maybe your caregivers no longer say positive things like "as soon as you're off chemotherapy" or "everything looks fine on that last scan."

Instead, they may recommend a new, more frequent course of treatment, or yet another round of tests, or exploratory surgery. When you ask your doctor about your progress, she no longer uses the word "cure." Now, it's "control of remission."

Your cancer has recurred. Or it is a different type of cancer, in a different part of your body; but for you, cancer survival means you're living with cancer that is chronic.

People can survive with chronic cancer for years; sometimes decades. I did find women who have been diagnosed two, three, four and more times than that with different cancers, over a span of many years. They never get beyond cancer, but they are living as well as possible with cancer.

But what happens when the cancer is back, or it never went away, and you know that you have only a limited time left?

None of us dies of cancer. We die of stroke, or heart attack, or, most often, pneumonia after being weakened by cancer.

Dying of cancer may not have been the ending you would have chosen for your life; yet it is not the worst way to go, either. There usually is little pain and disability until the very advanced stages. Cancer pain is something that can be controlled by various methods.

There will also be emotional pain, the pain of leaving the people you love and the anguish of dying with goals, hopes and dreams unfulfilled, but cancer is a disease that gives you time to say goodbye. And there will be the work of bringing your life to completion and of accepting the fact that you have come to the final season of your life.

Just as it was difficult and painful to accept that you have cancer, now you are faced with an even harsher reality: your cancer has returned and is now so widespread that you cannot survive.

Acceptance that death is not in the distant future but in a matter of months is a process.

You did not instantly accept the changes cancer brought to your life, and you cannot expect to accept your coming death with calm grace. Not yet, and perhaps not ever. Before acceptance for most people who know they are dying there are periods of:

Denial: It can't be happening. I feel well enough. I'm too young. There is so much I haven't seen yet, so much I haven't done!

I haven't had enough time!

Why me? Why not someone who's old, someone who doesn't have much to live for?

Depression: It's so unfair! I've worked so hard. I was just beginning to get somewhere. What have I done to deserve this? I might as well just lie down and die. Why prolong it?

Anger: I feel so angry. How could the doctor have missed finding it, until it was too late? Why isn't this treatment working? Why didn't they get it all, before? Why did they keep telling me "Don't worry! You'll be fine!" Now they say, "There's nothing more we can do for you." And I trusted them!

Fear: I am going to need people to do everything for me. To look after me. But what if they won't, or can't? I'm afraid of dying in pain. I'm most afraid of dying alone. Maybe it would be best for everyone if I just disappeared -- just took off. Then my family wouldn't have to watch me die. They'd be spared this misery, at least.

Linda is 33 and a graduate student, the woman who had to move in with her father after she learned she had advanced Hodgkin's.

Four years ago, she went to her doctor with what she thought was a cold she couldn't shake. He treated her for a persistent infection and tonsillitis for almost a year before diagnosing cancer.

When he told her the correct diagnosis, he added that she had perhaps six months to a year to live.

But Linda has now survived two years beyond that six months.

"When the doctor told me, I was just numb. I walked for hours, I don't remember where.

"For about two months, I denied it all. And then I was very angry. I felt like two people. The woman who is alive, and the woman who is dying. For a long time, I thought that acceptance would only come when I had realized or maybe resolved my own death. Now, I see that acceptance of your own death is a part of living, just like denial. It's daily."

Recently, Linda learned that her treatment is no longer working. Remission has ended. "I'm not God, so I don't really know anything other than to say I'm alive until I'm not. I go to my classes. I have written a pamphlet for newly diagnosed cancer patients, about the emotional side of cancer. Doing this, and talking to people about cancer, has helped me learn that people really do live their dying the same way they've lived their lives."

Some people find ways to live their final months that would not work for others. Linda chose to go to school for as long as possible. We each make our own path to acceptance just as, in earlier seasons in our lives, we mapped our individual routes to happiness or wealth or fulfilment.

Linda lives alone but she says she feels "very lucky. I have had a few central people in my life who have helped me talk this problem out. They taught me that life is worth fighting for."

Now near the end of her life, she says, "I feel more alive. I'm also more self-sufficient, even though I still worry about being alone at the end. My life goals have changed, even the day-to-day ones. My significant circle is now very small, by choice. I value my time. I've found value to my time."

She has done this by shifting her attention, from accomplishments she may never have the time to attain, to relationships here and now: "It's simply re-thinking what is really important, to me."

While you're grappling with depression, anger, fear and doubt, so are the people around you. If you have very young children, they recognize the turmoil without understanding the reason, and this uncertainty terrifies them.

The kindest gift you can give your children and everyone else who is losing you is the tools they need for their own grief and eventual recovery.

The end of grieving will not come for them until after your death, but you can help them now by telling them the truth.

Very young children see death literally, as a witch or a monster or a vicious animal such as a lion or tiger that comes in the night to eat them. For them, death is the subject of nightmares.

One way to tell children about your death without

terrorizing them is to explain that your body is very, very ill. It is not working right, and the doctors do not know how to fix it.

Your body is dying, so you can no longer live in it. Because of that, you must leave your body behind. If you believe in Heaven, describe where your spirit will go. If you do not, you may wish to say simply that you will go to a beautiful garden far away. Make it clear that, without your body, you cannot come back, and that no one can visit you there.

Do not tell a child that you are going to sleep, because she will be terrified to go to bed at night, and do not tell her you are going away.

She will keep expecting you to return.

Instead, tell her how very sad you are that you must leave her, but that you must go. You have no choice in this.

Tell your child that you will love her forever. Let her know that the sad feelings she is having now are okay to have and that these feelings of sadness or anger will gradually go away, but that you know she will always remember you.

Talk about the happy times you have had together. Remind her of special family days and joyous events. Make a memory book picture album together and write captions that tell where you were, what you did that day and why it made you happy.

Write her letters, or a journal, telling her you love her and all your hopes and dreams for her future. Write a letter to be saved and opened on the day she graduates, starts her first adult job, marries, has her own child.

Tell her now that you would do anything in the world to be able to stay, but that you can't.

And tell her that even though you can't be there to see her grow up, she will still be cared for by Daddy, or Grandma, or whomever you have chosen as her guardian.

Remind her of all the people who love her.

Reassure her that what is happening to you now will not happen to her.

In **Talking with Young Children about Death**, educator Hedda Bluestone Sharapan stresses the importance of being honest with children when you or someone you love is dying: "We need to remember that when there are unanswered questions (or unspoken ones) children will find their own fantasy explanations... If we try to hide our overwhelming sadness, children may wonder if we are sad or not -- and whether it's all right for them to be. Grieving together gives us the chance to offer each other comfort: 'We both feel sad, don't we?' 'You're not alone in how you feel.'

You will probably need to repeat these messages many times, because no one really hears and understands sad news the first time. The actual words you use are not important, if they are loving.

More important than what you say is that you have paid attention to your child's need to know; that you are not excluding her or him. By doing this, you show your child that you love them. Even though you can't be with her always, the memory of your caring will help her grow into a strong and loving person.

Younger children worry most about the loss of your maternal care and protection. Children older than five or six are more apt to be very angry and resentful ("How can you be doing this to me?) or to deny that it is happening for an extended period ("No, you're not going away. I won't let you!).

Grown children, like your parents, friends and your mate will also react in disbelief, anger and sorrow. And these are the times that we say, and may do, hurtful and thoughtless things. Much as you want to, you can't take their grief away. Each must cope with losing you in his or her own way.

For some this may mean disruptive behaviour in

class, for others stone-faced withdrawal or a new pensiveness.

Here are some things you can do to ease everyone's anguish, including your own:

Share your fears, hopes, dreams as well as your disappointments with the people you love. Why did you go out with your mate, that first time? When did you first realize that you love him or her? What things do you love most about him? What has your life together meant to you?

Have you told friends what you value in your relationship with them?

Or have your told your children what it was like to be pregnant with them, or awaiting their arrival if you adopted, and what their birth or your first meeting was like? What did you like and appreciate about them then? What are the characteristics and abilities you value in them now?

Says Hedda Bluestone Sharapan, "For instance, you might comment: 'I love your expressive eyes.' 'I admire the responsible attitude you have toward your homework.' 'I think your enthusiasm for sports is super.' "

"Tell you children what you enjoy doing with them... Don't focus on things you don't like." widely syndicated parenting expert Saf Lerman suggests in

Building a Child's Positive Self-Image. "Take time to let your children know that you are glad to be a parent, and, more specifically, glad to be their parent."

It also helps children to learn what you like and appreciate about yourself as a person and as a parent. For example, "What I like about myself as a mother is my good sense of humour and my joy in watching you children grow."

If your relationships are less than happy, now is the time to bring the problems out into the open and resolve them.

Are there leftover angers or resentments?

Talk about them.

Give your family the chance to forgive, and to be forgiven.

If you find it difficult to talk about your deepest feelings, write them down. Perhaps your children are too young, or your spouse is too lost in grief to hear what you have to say. One way to be sure they know is to write them letters.

Hedda Bluestone Sharapan also suggests making a memory book with notes and pictures of special moments and favourite things shared. By creating these memories, she writes, "We reaffirm for a child -

- and for us -- that the people we love go on living in our minds and that they will always be an important part of who we are now and who we grow up to be."

One woman, knowing she would not live long enough to be at her youngest daughter's wedding, put all her loving wishes and hopes for her daughter's future happiness into a letter to be kept in a safety deposit box until the wedding day.

Another, even more personal way to do this is to record your message.

Another loving thing you do for your family is get your affairs in order. Make (or update) your will. If there are things (like jewellery or a family heirloom) you want a specific person to have, give it to them now.

If you are a single parent, who have you chosen to raise your children? Have you arranged for a trust fund to provide for them? Make this provision in writing, with a lawyer.

It is best for your children if you choose people they are already close to and if they know what the arrangements are. The courts will honour this wish if the arrangement is uncontested in most areas.

If you do not choose a guardian, the courts will appoint one, meaning your children will lose you and their home and possibly be placed in foster care to await adoption -- added trauma for them.

Make decisions about where and how you wish to die. Most people still die in hospital, although there is a growing recognition that hospitals, with their emphasis on curing people, are generally not the best place to die in tranquillity and dignity.

In hospital, you may be alone much more than you want to be. In some, visiting is limited. Your children, grandchildren and pets may not be able to visit you.

In most, there is little privacy. Although you may be able to arrange to be left alone for a time, you must specifically request it, and it may not be granted.

There may be tests and other invasive medical procedures that are unpleasant. Also, hospitals are usually so short-staffed that you may receive very little emotional support and your family and friends may receive none.

Until recently, the only alternative was to die at home. Traditionally, surrounded by familiar people and possessions, people could die in their own bed. But we no longer live in extended families where there are people with the time to care for us.

Today, few people believe they have the option of dying at home, surrounded by family and friends and their caring support. Some families can manage it with the help of volunteers and visiting nurses and homemakers, but home care services are expensive and in short supply.

Another alternative is to die in a palliative care unit, also called hospice care.

A hospice is a place, sometimes your own home, but more often a separate care home or hospital ward, where you can die in dignity, surrounded by people who will work to make your life as good and as comfortable as possible for as long as possible, without any heroics at the end.

The philosophy behind hospice care is not to prolong life beyond the time when it is meaningful to you. Rather, hospice's primary goal is the comfort and emotional support of people and their families. This concern for the quality of life includes pain control.

Drugs for pain are usually most effective when used in combination and given continuously rather than given sporadically or only when pain becomes unbearable. It is possible to regulate these drugs so that you can be comfortable, and still be yourself, almost to your final moment.

Pain is increased when you are tense and when you fight it; and it is lessened when you accept it and try to think of something else. Remember, too, that pain is subjective. When it hurts, ask for pain relief, and if the medication you are given doesn't help you, tell your caregivers. Do not wait to ask for relief. The tension caused by mounting pain can only intensify it. Keep in mind that not all pain relievers work for everyone. Help your caregivers find the combination that allows you to be most comfortable.

Make your funeral arrangements. It has been your life, and now this is your death. Do you want cremation, or burial? A funeral, or a later Celebration of Life, or neither of these? Do you want to be buried, or cremated? If you own a cemetery plot, where is it? Make your choices and either make the arrangements (it is possible to pre-arrange and pre-pay a funeral) or put your desires in writing and be sure that your spouse and your executor or other responsible person knows of your choices.

For many of us, it is a great comfort knowing that a part of us will live on, giving the gift of a better life to someone we will never meet. Unfortunately, it's usually not possible for people who have cancer to donate their eyes or an organ after death because of the damage done by cancer and treatment. This may not be true for you. Your doctor will be able to tell you, or write for information to one of the organ donation societies in your country (find them online).

Novelist Robertson Davies has written that "... when

one person dies, a whole world of hope and memory and feeling dies with him." For the mate left behind, some of those memories and regrets remain as the afterglow of grief. Betty had died eight years ago, but her husband Woody couldn't let down his burden of regret for their three "not so good" years that came after more than thirty very good years together, for which he blamed only himself.

How did a good marriage turn sour in their 50s? They never talked about it.

They met when Woody was an army sergeant stationed in Florida waiting to be shipped overseas just as the United States entered World War II. Theirs was a wartime romance of brief meetings and long separations.

After his Army discharge, Betty and Woody bought a home and had two sons. She became a social worker, rising quickly in the civil service; he taught and then went into television management. They prospered.

Just five years before they planned to retire, Betty developed what seemed to be stomach flu.

Her doctor suspected a problem with her gall bladder, but during surgery it was discovered that she had cancer of the colon which had already spread to her liver.

Woody: "The surgery was in March. Betty was

feeling great a few days after her surgery and I went up to see her. She was sitting up in a chair looking real perky. I took her hand and I said, 'I've got some bad news, dear,' and she said, 'Oh, what?'

" 'Well,' I said, 'they discovered you have a tumour on your liver.' And she just sat there, kind of staring at me. Finally, she said, 'My God, what have I done to you?'

"Not, 'poor me' or bewailing her fate, but it was me that she was thinking of. I broke down. I had to get up and I walked to the bathroom and I confess I shed a few tears. When I came back, she was still dry-eyed and she tried to cheer me up.

"She seemed really well for the first month after surgery. But then she progressively got weaker.

"During her four-month illness, I was able to care for her at home. I learned to cook, after a fashion and did things I never dreamed possible.

"Finally, in July, it got to the point where I just couldn't do it any longer, as much as she wanted to be at home and as much as I wanted to care for her. So, I took her back to hospital. She died there five days later.

"Have you ever wished that you could back up and do something all over again, just wipe the board clean? I have felt that way so may times about my relationship with Betty. We were close, but we had our problems. She had wanted to adopt another child, a little girl. She really wanted that, but I didn't. Now I wish so much that we had. We were married for 33 years and I would say we were happy, but I found it difficult to really sit down and talk about things that are personally important. About how I felt.

"Just as an example, it was extremely difficult for me to discuss sex with Betty. This was stupid of me but it was true. I didn't tell her I loved her as much as I should have. I always assumed that she knew and you know, if I could live it all over again, it would have been an entirely different relationship.

"We never really talked about her illness. I know that she knew that it was terminal and, of course, I knew and I guess lurking in the back of our minds was that hope against hope that maybe she would be lucky. We never discussed that she was terminal.

"One time, she said to me, 'You know, Woody, you're going to outlive me!' and I just pooh-poohed it. I wish I had talked to her about it--about the future.

"But in the last weeks we did talk about the good times that we had had and some of the wonderful, funny things that happened to us over the years. And we talked about our boys. I think in these talks we became very close. But we never talked about her death -- right or wrong?

"Once, she asked me if I thought we would ever be able to have sex again. I said, 'Why, of course, just as soon as you are physically able to.' I said that even though we both knew by then that it was terminal.

"I didn't cry until a month after her death. I think that friends probably did more to help me than anything else. In the years since Betty died, loneliness has been my biggest problem. Now I have retired, and I guess the fact that I keep busy with hobbies and travel have helped."

Heartbreakingly, he still feels guilt and shame for what went wrong in their marriage, even though every marriage works (or doesn't) because of the choices and actions of two people, not one. Their final weeks together were close and loving, perhaps among the best times of their marriage.

Yet he lives wracked by regrets.

Woody says he would give anything to have a second chance with Betty. He never told her this. Now, he wonders if she knew.

Any crisis, particularly an on-going health crisis,

tends to bring out the worst, but also the best, in people. Trauma forces us to either cope and grow in resilience, or to not cope (for example, by trying to hide out in denial) and so be weakened in character and spirit.

Not only will some of your anger and frustration be vented towards the people you look to for love and support, but also some of their negative emotions will be dumped upon you.

Relationships that were troubled aren't likely to bloom now, when you are seriously ill, even though time to make things better is running out.

A marriage that was not truly intimate and happy, where most of the sharing of common interests was with other people, won't suddenly become the marriage you may have always wanted but never, for whatever reason, managed to build. And no matter how close you and your mate have been, no one person can ever be everything you need.

While you are dying, your world will narrow, and it will become increasingly hard to maintain your relationships.

But you will need your closest friends, and some of these may be new friends, as much as you need your mate.

As in every other stage of life, the quality of the final

days of your life really is up to you. You can choose to have less pain, just as you can choose to find joy in the small things, like sunlight shafting through your window, or a jar of pussywillows, or the antics of a kitten, simple things you might not have noticed for years.

Only you can make the choice to give up anger and guilt and sadness for what might have been and concentrate instead on what can be done now to banish despair.

"This is not a time for lamenting, but for intense living," says Doctor Elizabeth Latimer, director of palliative care services at Hamilton Civic Hospital in Ontario. "One man told me the last six months of his life were better than the previous 60 years. That is often true." In this season of your life you can speak your mind, saying what you always wished you could say. It is also a time of asking for what you want, reviewing your life and finding what was good there, and renewing or intensifying your faith, in God, or in people and the continuity of life.

Now, at the end of her life, Linda no longer attends classes, but the friends she made when she went back to school are the friends who visit her in hospice. Her world has become the boundaries of her room, but the visits of friends sustain her. Through them she lives in the world she chose for the last years of her life. She did not fulfil the dream of earning her degree, but that doesn't matter. There is no more need to strive, and no more need to fight the disease. There is only the need to love, and let be.

"In this time, I've really gotten to know myself" she wrote. "Things I used to take little notice of now seem very important and vivid. These last months, I have truly been happy. I wake up every morning to a new day, not an alarm clock."

TEN

Life is the Best Gift

Back in 1980, I asked "Why me?" Why did I have cancer?

Today, when I wonder "Why me?" the question is really, "Why have I survived when there are now family members and friends whose survival was far too short a time?"

If it were simply a matter of hope or faith or being positive, then surely seminal thinker Barbara Ward, marathon hero and humanitarian Terry Fox, reggae singer and composer Bob Marley, musician and composer George Harrison, politicians Jack Layton and Hubert Humphrey, actors Ingrid Bergman, John Wayne and Humphrey Bogart, novelist Margaret Laurence and so many others would still be among us.

Why do we survive?

And how do we survive?

What does survival mean?

What does it mean to live with cancer and live beyond cancer?

Those were the questions that started me on this journey of discovery. One of the things I learned from the women I sought out to ask these questions is that it is not really hope or even courage alone that bring about survival. It isn't any one thing that any of us can name.

One day, science may have more to offer us – prevention, cures -- but until that day, we (being human) need to make sense of our cancer experiences.

Cancer needs to mean something, in our lives.

Survival needs to mean something; to turn out to have been worth all the effort it took to get here.

We go on, living one day at a time, and after a while the days stack up into months and the months to years. The morning comes when we realize it has been five years since treatment, and there has been no recurrence. While the doctors and the rest of the medical community see something magical in this five-year goal-post, really there isn't. We who have had cancer know it could come back, at any time, and that we must learn to live with this knowledge.

Feel the fear, and keep living well despite this.

Each of us becomes a survivor not when we get to that five-year survival mark, but in the very moment of diagnosis.

That is the moment when cancer tilts our world, changing everything.

In becoming a survivor and talking to other women who are survivors, I have learned that the shock-and-awe pain of cancer fades, with time, but the strengths and growth gained do not fade.

When I look back at the woman I was before cancer, I marvel at her foolish belief in our cultural myths and at her childish irresponsibility for her physical well-being. It surprises me that she could have been so naive, so ready to believe what others said and disbelieve herself.

She was a child-woman, not yet an adult, not really. She'd built up some resilience in life, some coping skills, but these were modest coming up against the demands cancer trauma presents.

It shocks me to remember how I took my good health and good fortune for granted, believing that anything that might go wrong with my body would be minor and could easily be fixed by doctors; that major things could not go wrong, not with my body or in my life, for no reason except that I was young, healthy, middle class, average.

It shames me to admit that, at age 29, I still believed in the fairytale ending, the happily-ever-after, finding the wondrous career and even more wondrous man I thought were simply my due. I marvel at how I could have been so unaware of my own health and needs; so blind to the health and needs of others and our world.

I am more realistic now, I think, more mature and more responsible. But the child-woman of years ago is not so different from the person I am today. It would be nice to think that I am more tolerant, more patient, more compassionate -- a kinder and better version of myself all round. I am, sometimes. I am much the same person, but my life is different, richer, fuller, and my appreciation for it is no longer a matter of course. I no longer take life nor the people in my life for granted.

In these years, I have come to see the frailty of life, the vulnerabilities of other people and within myself. I have learned about trusting the woman I see in the mirror. I can accept myself, as I am now. I have learned to build on strengths.

Women told me of the richness of their lives, after and beyond cancer. I learned from them that survival can be anything you want and need it to be. Survival truly is a second chance to live, a chance to change the rules you used to live by, a chance to redefine who you need to be and who and what you need to include in your life. It is a rebirth.

And I have learned that it is not possible to keep all the promises we make when we are threatened and afraid. To live life on a natural high, drinking in each golden moment, is unnatural. There are still bad times, still sad times, still the days when I am insensitive and afraid.

Still days when I am angry.

Still days when I cry.

But there are more days when I am so much happier, so much more alive than I or most other people ever expect someone who had cancer to be. I also know that I can stand some pain, some tough times, and I will not be crushed.

And if cancer comes back again? Oh God -- but, if it does? Then I will survive, again. Not without anger and tears. But also, not without faith in myself and in my support system.

This time would be different, because I know I made it once. With help, I can make it again.

There are women, like the women you have met in this book, whose outpouring of caring and kindness and insights have enriched my survival.

They are a source of empathy and compassion that is there for all of us to find. There are women like us everywhere now.

Also, I know my mate would help me. My sister introduced us.

Soon, I was seeing him almost every evening and it occurred to me that being with him was becoming very important to me. The time had come to tell him about the cancer, but that also meant the risk of losing what was becoming more than friendship.

I put it simply, explaining that I'd had cancer and two mastectomies, but that I was well now. As I spoke, he stared at his hands. Soon after, he mumbled good night and left.

He did not call the next day, or the day after that. I longed to know his reaction, but I forced myself not to call. I wished I didn't care so much. A week went by. No call.

Finally, early one evening he phoned and half an hour later was at my door. We cooked spaghetti, he made the salad and as we ate we talked about friends and work. I gathered my courage to ask him how he felt about the cancer. About me.

"I thought about it all the time," he said. "At work, with friends, when I tried to read, all the time. And the one thing I kept thinking was that I should just walk away. But also, I kept thinking of you. Once I realised I would rather have five minutes with you, any five minutes, than the rest of my life alone, then I knew I had to deal with it."

What I did not know until much later is that Wayne's closest friend through high school, Mike, had died of cancer when he was 20.

Accepting that I'd had cancer but that I was surviving was not easy for him, and it didn't happen in one evening of talking. He has had to face all the fears felt by the mates of people with cancer. Two years ago, there was another lump, between my breasts. He was with me during the examination, the biopsy, and when we learned that this time, it was just another harmless lump. In every sense, he shares in my survival.

"It's not so bad," he said, the first time he saw my changed body. "Not really so much different than these." He pointed to pencil line scars on his shoulders and chest, the lingering reminders of being wild and free on a motorcycle when he was eighteen. "It makes no difference to me. It's just another part of you," he added tenderly, pulling me into his embrace. "All of you is beautiful to me."

INTIMACY

With him, I have learned about acceptance; that it is a vital part of love.

Four hours after our son was born in hospital, while Wayne was home for a shower and breakfast, our baby lay nestled between my breasts, asleep. A nurse looked in on us.

"Ah, what a lovely sight," she said in a soft Scottish accent. He was lovely, amazing, perfect. Like any other new mother, I admired him tremendously but wondered where he had come from and who had assigned me to see to his needs. At first, he seemed like some other woman's child, some healthy young mother like my roommate, not mine. I marvelled that my scared body could produce a flawless baby.

My new child and I had only one bittersweet moment, during our first few days together, when another nurse appeared to announce, "Time you learn to breastfeed him, Mrs Johnson!" I told her that would be impossible.

"Now, dear, we all find it a little bit difficult at first . . ." I interrupted to suggest, not very nicely, that she go and check my chart. She didn't come back and that was the last mention of breastfeeding. Jesse nuzzled at my reconstructed breasts a few times, but of course there was no milk there. He was allergic to goats' milk, so we gave up our suspicions about the benefits of formula and he thrived.

I'm sorry Jesse and I missed the experience of breast-feeding, but we cuddled skin to skin as he drank from bottles. I do not believe we could possibly have become more closely bonded if I could have breastfed. Today he is my special reward for having survived.

The word "survive" means to outlive or outlast. I do not think that I conquered cancer. I do believe that, with help and love and kindness from many people, I have outlasted cancer.

I met many women who have done this, and have gone beyond mere survival to restructure and reinvent lives that are more meaningful for them and those they love. These women continue to inspire me.

From their stories, I have learned about pain and loss and loneliness, that these are part of everyone's life. And I have re-learned about the beauty of life, about those quiet moments when you discover that you can accept your changed self, that cancer is a part of your life but not the definition of your life, that within your changed body there is a strong, whole woman.

Survival is measured in quality, not in quantity. Some of the women I found and you have met in this book have died. As I wrote, I thought often of them, particularly of Cheryl. I remember the way she curled her feet under her to sit in the corner of my chesterfield, her voice, her smile. I think of what I am doing today, right now, and wonder if she would enjoy it too. I wish she were here.

Today, I know I want to live, not only to get ahead in my career; not for status; not because of duties that must be met and promises that must be kept; not even for goals and dreams and longings and the time to maybe fulfil some of them, but for now, for this moment.

I realise that, for some probably unknowable reason, I am one of the lucky ones, a survivor. The loving husband and healthy child I once thought I'd lost forever are a reality today. To be alive, right now, is the best gift I have ever received.

From women and from my own heart I have learned that you must trust your feelings. Trust yourself. Strive for your survival, and for the survival of our earth. Are there are toxic wastes buried in your neighbourhood? Do you know how safe your water is? Do you urge friends to stop smoking and to drink in moderation (because not doing this also raises your risk of cancer)?

Have you worked to ban junk food from your child's school cafeteria, stopped using "edible petroleum products," safely disposed of garden pesticides rather than use them? Learn what you can to help prevent cancer!

We who have healed ourselves and our families must work to heal our world. Otherwise, cancer, not survival, is the certain future for us all.

Together, we are stronger than any mutant cell; our lives richer and more meaningful than the mere reaction to what the cells within our bodies may be doing, or not doing, right now.

At some point in the future, we will certainly be able to cure cancer – and at some future date, surely, we will eradicate it. Until then, we can't sit back and wait for 'doctors' or 'research' or 'the experts' or 'the drug companies' to come up with answers – we who are the cancer survivors and cancer veterans must do this. For ourselves, for the people we care about, for other women.

Our lives – and everything these lives can be – depend on it.

We live as fully as we can, for as long as we can, with cancer as just one of those tough things that befalls real people, in the real world. While we did not choose this path, we can choose how we will travel on it and, ultimately, beyond it.

Dedication

This book is dedicated to all cancer survivors, and everyone who loves them and cares for them.

And in memory of Betty Wentzy, Woody Wentzy, Ken Fieber and Cheryl Alber.

"Those whom we love go on living in our hearts so long as we live"

-Havelock Ellis, in his last letter to his lover, Francoise Lafitte-Cyon.

INTIMACY

Acknowledgments

Surviving cancer and writing a book about that survival have little in common, except for one all-important aspect. You can neither create your survival nor write a book without the help and patient encouragement of a host of other people. To this wonderfully generous support group, I offer my heartfelt gratitude:

To the women who shared their experiences, both their pain and their triumphs, to help me, other women and the people who care about us and care for us understand the personal toll cancer takes, I am deeply grateful. Their strength and courage helped sustain me in this task, and serve as a continuing inspiration in my own life.

For statistics and other background material on cancer, I am indebted to The Canadian Cancer Society National Office, Statistics Canada, The

American Cancer Society National Headquarters, the Department of Health & Human Services of the (American) National Cancer Institute and Cancer Research Campaign in England. I particularly thank Jane R Tom, Research Fellow in Cancer Statistics, Cancer Research Campaign in London and Edwin Silverberg, Researcher at National Headquarters, American Cancer Society in New York City for their assistance in getting the statistics and understanding them.

Rose Kushner's pioneering book, **Why Me?** (now titled **Alternatives**), was a source of needed information as well as a model of competent, careful journalism. For helping to shape my thinking on death and dying, I am grateful to Elisabeth Kubler-Ross, M.D., one of the first caregivers in our era to point out that the most important skill in healing is listening.

The trail-blazing work of Alfred Kinsey and the more recent findings of William Masters, M.D. and Virginia Johnson formed the firm foundation of my understanding of human sexuality, and the work of Sheila Kitzinger and Bernie Zilbergeld, Ph.D. has added walls and windows to my understanding of how couples relate.

In making the links between sexuality, body image, self image and cancer, the research findings and insights generously shared by the following caregivers and experts were of immeasurable help, for which I thank them: Joy Rogers, R.N. and Mary L.S. Vachon, R.N., Ph.D., both of The Clarke Institute of Psychiatry in Toronto; Clement Persaud, Ph.D. of Canadore College in North Bay, Ontario; Leslie R. Schover, Ph.D. and Andrew C. von Eschenbach, M.D., both of M.D. Anderson Hospital at the University of Texas, who kindly allowed me to read their work on cancer and sexuality while in press; Leonard R. Derogatis, Ph.D., of the Johns Hopkins University School of Medicine; Judi Johnson, R.N., Ph.D., North Memorial Medical Center, Robbinsdale, Minnesota; Pepper Schwartz, Ph.D., University of Washington in Seattle, John Lamont, M.D., McMaster University, Hamilton, Ontario and Joseph LoPiccolo, Ph.D., School of Medicine, State University of New York at Stony Brook.

I also thank Walter Rider, M.B., of Princess Margaret Hospital Toronto, who cared for people with cancer for over three decades with gentleness, tact, generosity of spirit and a delightfully dry sense of humour. His colleague, M. Vera Peters, M.D., kindly shared her research findings on pregnancy and cancer, and helped ease our worries during our own pregnancy.

Albert Bandura, Ph.D., of Stanford University shared

his findings and insights on caring for people with heart disease and answered my questions about possible implications of his work for people with cancer; J. Michael Dreger, M.D., F.R.C.S.(C) of Toronto added to my knowledge of breast cancer and reconstruction, and author-educator Saf Lerman, M.D. Ed. of Boston gave thoughtful answers to my questions on parenting.

Cathy Jenison, R.N., M.Ed. of South Dakota State University was both a caring friend and counsellor who helped me see that grieving is a way of growing.

Kathleen V. Cairns, Ph.D., of the University of Calgary has been a source of limitless inspiration and guidance. She shared knowledge, insights, and research I would not otherwise have been able to read and has been an enthusiastic supporter throughout this project. I am also grateful to Michael Barrett, Ph.D., of The Sex Information and Education Council of Canada and University of Toronto, for his help and encouragement, and for introducing me to Kathy Cairns.

Among the most enthusiastic health advocates for women I found are nurses.

In often difficult working environments, during long hours, many nurses continue to perform wonders in helping women adjust to the changes cancer brings.

For adding to my education and understanding, I thank these nurses: Trisha Bach of Minneapolis; Kaye Meek of Toronto; Kathy Smith and June Scruton, both of Henderson General Hospital in Hamilton; Marilyn J. Deachman at Princess Margaret Hospital in Toronto, and Judith Leyden, who cared for me at Brookings Hospital in South Dakota.

I am also grateful to June Scruton, Kathy Smith and Carol Passmore for reading the manuscript and offering their suggestions and constructive criticism.

I thank Joan Webber of the Ministry of Community and Social Services in Toronto who explained adoption policies.

For telling me of the advances being made in the science and art of prosthetics, I am very grateful to Bill Sauter, C.P.O.(c) of The Hugh Macmillan Centre in Toronto

The Ontario Arts Council gave me a grant that helped in completing the research, for which I am grateful.

Ms. Magazine, Toronto Star and The Body Politic initially and later Healthsharing, The Complete Mother and A Friend Indeed all published notices that helped me find women to answer the questionnaire.

I thank Jane Selley, of The Palliative Care Foundation

in Toronto, for information on hospice care and pain control for people who are dying.

Friends in the States and in Canada, whose kindness and compassion sustained me in my own recovery and in writing this book, are Woody Wentzy and Nancy Helgerson, my two lifelines during my own darkest days, and Pat Eich, Kathy and Mike Clites, Darla Solem, Gary Stagliano, Joyce Lampson, Pat McCorkle, Tim Shank, Jan and Dave Sanford, Ruth Breazeale, Renee Silberman, Carol Passmore, Diane Reitz, Barbara Walker and Jeff Froud. Other friends who have pitched in to help are Bob Holzman, who took my cover photo for the original print edition of this book and Pat and Jim Kerkmaz, who tracked down a needed fact as we faced deadline.

R.A. Nelson, my journalism teacher at Wheeling (Illinois) High School, was the first person to suggest I might, someday, be published and I thank him for that leap of faith, the mark of every good teacher.

Most of all, I thank the extraordinarily kind and encouraging person who read and re-read the manuscript, listened, helped and supported me for the past year of writing; the person who has given me so much that has shaped and improved this work as well as my life, my best friend, Wayne Johnson. He is the one most responsible for keeping me on track, even when I thought I should give it all up to raise dachshunds or maybe sell hand-knit sweaters.

Without Wayne and our son, Jesse, my survival might have been possible, but it would have been less meaningful and a lot less joyous.

- JEJ

THANK YOU for reading. If you would like to know more about my other books, please visit

www.crimsonhillbooks.com

Made in the USA
Columbia, SC
10 March 2018